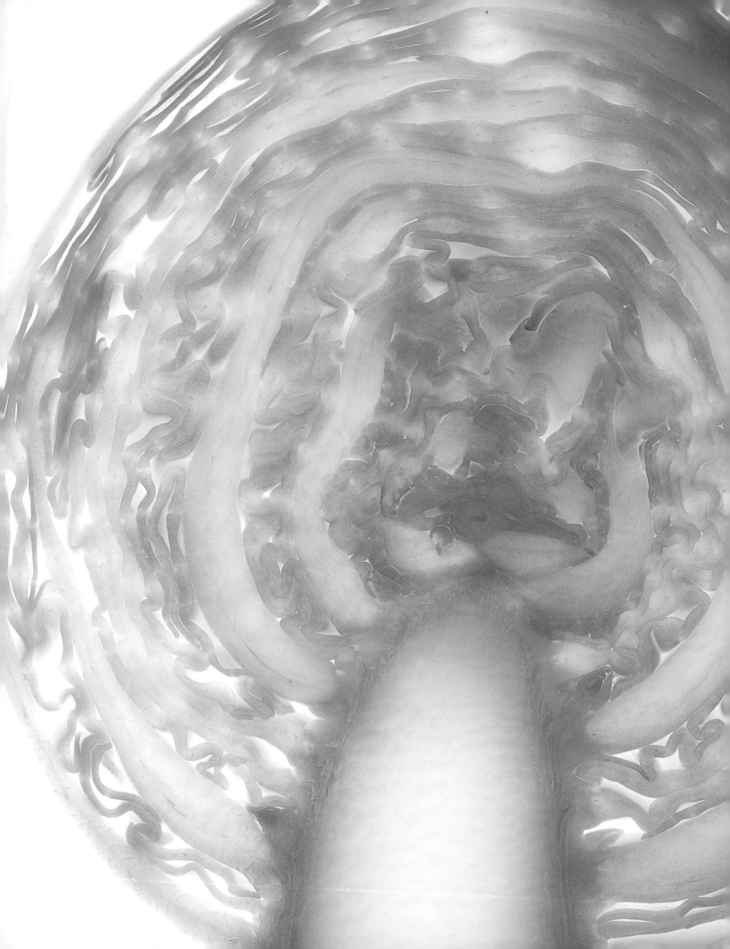

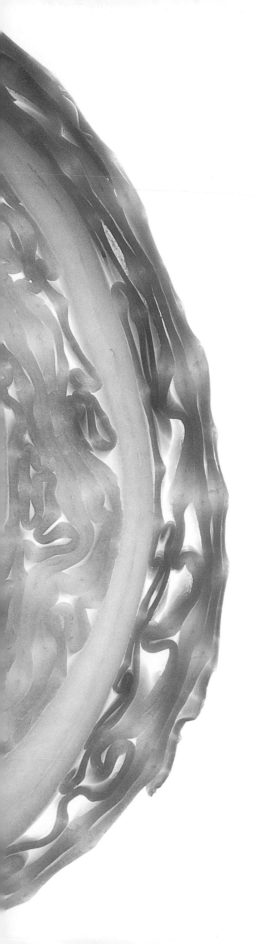

The YOGA Cookbook

Vegetarian Food for Body and Mind

Recipes from the Sivananda Yoga Vedanta Centers

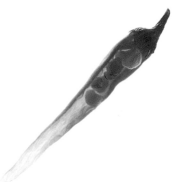

A Fireside Book
Published by Simon & Schuster

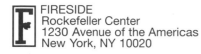

FIRESIDE
Rockefeller Center
1230 Avenue of the Americas
New York, NY 10020

FIRESIDE and colophon are registered trademarks
of Simon & Schuster Inc.

Designed by Sara Mathews

Printed and bound in Hong Kong

10 9 8 7 6 5

Library of Congress Cataloging-in-Publication Data is available.

ISBN 0-684-85641-7

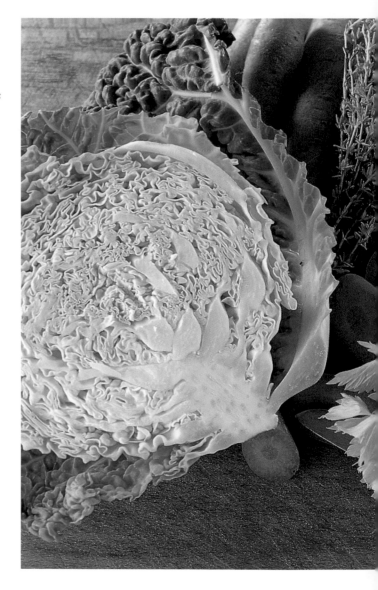

Publisher's note
This publication contains the opinions and ideas of Sivananda Yoga Vedanta Centers and is designed to provide useful advice to the reader on the subject matter covered. The publisher and author specifically disclaim any responsibility for any liability, loss or risk which may be claimed or incurred as a consequence, directly or indirectly, of the use of any of the contents of this publication.

Acknowledgements
Gaia Books would like to thank:
Felicity Jackson, Beverly LeBlanc, and Mary Pickles; home economists: Anne Sheasby, Angela Bogginao, and Steven Wheeler, and all those who tested the recipes; assistant to Carol Tennant: Kate Jay; models: Naya and Tejas; design assistants: Phil Gamble and Matt Moate; Crown Publishers for permission to reproduce quotes from The Complete Illustrated Book of Yoga *by Swami Vishnu-devananda copyright © 1960, 1988 by the Julian Press, Inc.*

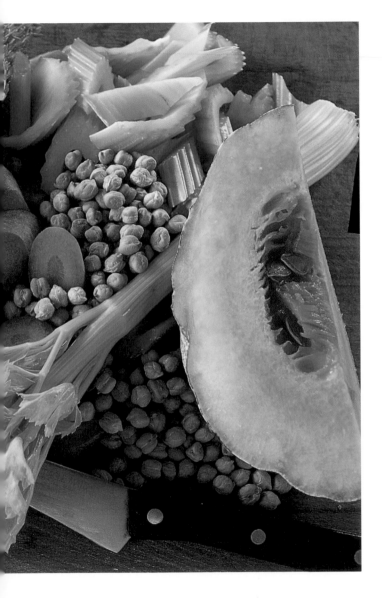

CONTENTS

The Sivananda Yoga Centers would like to thank:
Shakti Warwick (New York) for inspiring, writing, and compiling recipes for the first draft of this book; Shanti Smith (London) for doing the second draft and for developing the recipes into a publishable form; Uma Miller (Quebec) for compiling the Sivananda Cookbook from which many of the recipes were taken; Prema Venugopalan for the South Indian Bandara spread; Nigel Walker, Swami Radhapriyananda, Swami Gayatriananda, Ganesha, Kamala, Prema and Dattatreya, and so many others for contributing recipes; Jaya and Padmavati for organizing, Poorna and her team of dedicated Karma Yogis for testing, and all the students of the London Sivananda Yoga Centre for their patience in allowing the recipes to be tested on them.

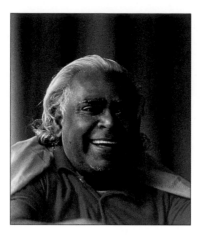

The Sivananda Yoga Vedanta Centers are a worldwide network of teaching facilities with international headquarters in Val Morin, Quebec, Canada. Founded by Swami Vishnu-devananda, recognized as one of the foremost authorities on Hatha and Raja Yoga, the purpose of the centers is to promote the teaching of the ancient science of yoga.

A native of South India, Swamiji (as he was popularly known) arrived in the West in 1957, after being sent by his teacher, Swami Sivananda, with the words "people are waiting." Dedicating his life to the cause of peace, both as inner discipline and on a global level, Swamiji realized that today, more than any other time in history, people are facing daily stresses and tensions beyond their control. He had a vision of how the age-old techniques of yoga could be used to solve many of the pressing problems of modern life, such as ill health, stress, personal alienation, and even war.

Swamiji synthesized the ancient wisdom of yoga into five principles, upon which he based his *The Complete Illustrated Book of Yoga*. Several years later he followed with *Meditation and Mantras*, one of the most complete sourcebooks available. He wrote a commentary on the ancient scripture, "Hatha Yoga Pradipika" and was the inspiration behind both *The Book of Yoga* and *Yoga Mind & Body*.

Swami Vishnu-devananda left his body in November 1993. Now there are 25 Sivananda Yoga Vedanta centers and ashrams, with many other affiliated centers and teachers, around the world.

Ashram Addresses

Sivananda Ashram Yoga Camp
8th Avenue, Val Morin
Quebec J0T 2R0, CANADA
Tel: (819) 322-3226 Fax: (819) 322-5876
email: hq@sivananda.org

Sivananda Ashram
Yoga Ranch Colony
PO Box 195, Budd Road
Woodbourne, NY 12788
Tel: (914) 434-9242 Fax: (914) 434-1032
email: YogaRanch@sivananda.org

Sivananda Ashram Yoga Retreat
PO Box N7550, Nassau, BAHAMAS
Tel: (242) 363-2902 Fax: (242) 363-3783
email: Nassau@sivananda.org

**Sivananda Yoga Vedanta
Dhanwanthari Ashram**
PO Neyyar Dam,
Thiruvanthapuram Dt.
Kerala 695 576, INDIA
Tel: (0471) 272-093
email: YogaIndia@sivananda.org

Sivananda Ashram Yoga Farm
14651 Ballantree Lane, Comp. 8
Grass Valley, CA 95949
Tel: (916) 272-9322 Fax: (916) 477-6054
email: YogaFarm@sivananda.org

Sivananda Kutir
(near Siror Bridge)
P.O. Netala, Uttara Kashi Dt.
(Himalayas) U.P. 249 193, INDIA
Tel: (01374) 2624

Center Addresses

AUSTRALIA
Sivananda Yoga Vedanta Centre
40 Ninth Avenue
Katoomba N.S.W. 2780
Tel: (2) 47 823245 Fax: (2) 47824185
email: SivanandaYogaBlueMts@Bigpond.com

AUSTRIA
Sivananda Yoga Vedanta Zentrum
Rechte Wienzeile 29-3-9
A-1040 Vienna
Tel: (01) 586-3453 Fax: (01) 587-1551
email: vienna@sivananda.org

CANADA
Sivananda Yoga Vedanta Center
5178 St Lawrence Blvd
Montreal, Quebec H2T 1R8
Tel: (514) 279-3545 Fax: (514) 279-3527
email: Montreal@sivananda.org

Sivananda Yoga Vedanta Center
77 Harbord Street
Toronto, Ontario M5S 1G4
Tel: (416) 966-9642 Fax: (416) 966-1378
email: Toronto@sivananda.org

FRANCE
Centre de Yoga Sivananda Vedanta
123 Boulevard Sebastopol
F-75002 Paris
Tel: (01) 40-26-77-49
Fax: (01) 42-33-51-97
email: Paris@sivananda.org

GERMANY
Sivananda Yoga Vedanta Zentrum
Steinheilstr. 1
D-80333 Munich
Tel: (089) 52-44-76 / 52-17-35
Fax: (089) 52-91-28
email: Munich@sivananda.org

Sivananda Yoga Vedanta Zentrum
Schmiljanstr. 24
D-12161 Berlin
Tel: (030) 8599 9799
Fax: (030) 8599 9797
email: Berlin@sivananda.org

INDIA
Sivananda Yoga Vedanta
Nataraja Centre
52 Community Centre, East of Kailash
New Delhi 110 065
Tel: (011) 648-0869 Fax: (011) 645-3962
email: Delhi@sivananda.org

Sivananda Yoga Vedanta Centre
37/1929, West Fort, Airport Road
Thiruvananthapuram, Kerala 695 023
Tel: (0471) 450-942 Fax: (0471) 451-776

Sivananda Yoga Vedanta Centre
A-9, 7th Main Rd
Thiruvalluvavar Nagar, Thiruvanmiyur
Chennai (Madras) 600 041
Tel: (044) 490-1626
email: Madras@sivananda.org

ISRAEL
Sivananda Yoga Vedanta Centre
6 Lateris St, Tel Aviv 64166
Tel: (03) 691-6793 Fax: (03) 696-3939
email: TelAviv@sivananda.org

SPAIN
Centro de Yoga Sivananda Vedanta
Calle Eraso 4
E-28028 Madrid
Tel: (91) 361-5150 Fax: (91) 361-5194
email: Madrid@sivananda.org

SWITZERLAND
Centre de Yoga Sivananda Vedanta
1 Rue de Minoteries
CH-1205 Geneva
Tel/Fax: (022) 328-0328
email: Geneva@sivananda.org

URUGUAY
Asociacion de Yoga Sivananda
Acevedo Diaz 1523
11200 Montevideo
Tel: (02) 401-09-29 / 401-66-85
Fax: (02) 400-73-88
email: Montevideo@sivananda.org

UNITED KINGDOM
Sivananda Yoga Vedanta Centre
51 Felsham Road
London SW15 1AZ
Tel: (0181) 780-0160
Fax: (0181) 780-0128
email: siva@dial.pipex.com

UNITED STATES
Sivananda Yoga Vedanta Center
1246 Bryn Mawr, Chicago, IL 60660
Tel: (312) 878-7771 Fax: (312) 878-7527
email: Chicago@sivananda.org

Sivananda Yoga Vedanta Center
243 West 24th Street
New York, NY 10011
Tel: (212) 255-4560 Fax: (212) 727-7392
email: NewYork@sivananda.org

Sivananda Yoga Vedanta Center
1200 Arguella Blvd
San Francisco, CA 94122
Tel: (415) 681-2731 Fax: (415) 681-5162
email: SanFrancisco@sivananda.org

Sivananda Yoga Vedanta Center
1746 Abbot Kinney Blvd
Venice (Los Angeles), CA 90291
Tel: (310) 822-9642 Fax: (310) 301-4214
email: LosAngeles@sivananda.org

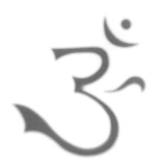

INTRODUCTION

Yogis believe
"the expression of the spirit increases in proportion to the
development of the body and mind in which it is encased.
Therefore, yoga prescribes methods to train and develop
the physical body and mind."

Swami Vishnu-devananda,
The Complete Illustrated Book of Yoga

The physical body is seen as an instrument, or vehicle, for the soul on its journey toward perfection. Just like other vehicles, this body/car has specific requirements which must be fulfilled for it to function smoothly and supply the optimum mileage. These requirements are the five yogic principles: proper exercise; proper breathing; proper relaxation; proper diet; and positive thinking and meditation.

Proper exercise acts as a lubricating routine. In yoga, physical exercises called asanas (the Sanskrit word means "steady pose") help to keep the joints, muscles, and other parts of the body functioning properly by increasing circulation and flexibility.

Proper breathing aids the body in connecting to its battery, the solar plexus, where tremendous potential energy is stored. When tapped through specific yoga breathing techniques, known as pranayama, this energy is released for physical and mental rejuvenation in the body.

Proper relaxation cools down the system like the radiator of a car does. When the body and mind are continually overworked, their efficiency diminishes. Relaxation is Nature's way of recharging the body and mind.

Proper diet provides the correct type of fuel. The body gets the energy it needs to work, grow, and maintain itself from the prana (vital energy), air, water, and food. The yogic diet is a vegetarian one, consisting of pure, natural foods that promote good health and optimum vitality.

Positive thinking and meditation puts you in control. Just as any vehicle requires an intelligent driver, the body needs a balanced mind. Regular meditation helps to clear and focus your mind and improve your ability to concentrate. Positive thinking will purify the intellect and help you to begin to experience wisdom and inner peace.

The Yogic Diet

This cookbook is concerned with the basic tenets of a "proper" yogic diet, traditionally a lactovegetarian one, consisting of grains, legumes, fruits, vegetables, nuts, seeds, and dairy products. As well as being simple, natural, and wholesome, this diet takes into account the subtle effect food has on the mind and the prana.

The question of whether humans are meant to be vegetarians is a topic that has been discussed by everyone from philosophers to anatomists. As far as health is concerned, meat is high in cholesterol and uric acid, as well as additives and preservatives—all of which contribute to a multitude of diseases. A primarily meat diet has been found to be a major contributor to such modern problems as high blood pressure, heart attacks, hardening of the arteries, arthritis, and gout. Excess uric acid lodged in the joints contributes to arthritis, while arteries clogged with cholesterol and other fatty deposits decrease the flow of blood to the brain, contributing to senility and raised blood pressure.

As if this is not bad enough, we are reminded that the meat business is run like a modern factory—cattle are seen as only so much saleable poundage. While on the hoof, animals are loaded up with megadoses of antibiotics to prevent illness (and loss of profits). Much of the residue of these hormones and antibiotics is left in the cells of the animals and, consequently, goes into the consumer's system. It is also interesting to note that even the most dedicated of meat-eaters in the West would shy away from eating a carnivorous animal, such as a cat or a dog. Perhaps this aversion is natural. As all energy originates from the sun, we instinctively realize the closer to the source we eat, the more potent is that energy.

The many physical reasons for being a vegetarian do not need to be discussed in detail here. Let it suffice to say animal protein is not necessary for good health. There are many other sources of protein, such as legumes, nuts, and seeds, as well as better vegetable sources of carbohydrates, fats, fiber, vitamins, and minerals—all of the nutrients we strive to access in our food. Having said that, let us turn to the psychological and spiritual basis for vegetarianism.

The animal world, for the most part, is a round of slaughter—the stronger or more cunning killing the weaker to survive, until they are devoured by an even mightier opponent. The difference with human beings is that we are endowed with intellect and free will, so we possess the ability to side-step a portion of this cycle and live in harmony with other life forms rather than in contest with them. The law of karma, which may be summarized as "for every action there is an equal and opposite reaction," is inexorable, unrelenting, and immutable. The that you inflict upon others will rebound upon you, and the happiness you radiate to another will come back to you, adding to your own happiness.

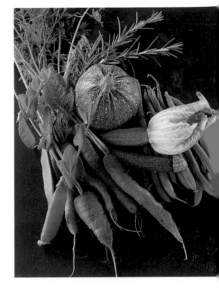

"By the purity of food, follows the purification of the inner nature."

Swami Sivananda

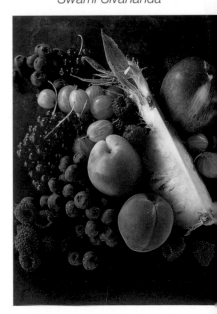

"Shortly after I began taking classes at the Sivananda Yoga Vedanta Center in America, I read The Complete Illustrated Book of Yoga by Swami Vishnu-devananda. Much of it was eye-opening to me, especially the chapter on the "Natural Diet of Man" (which I assumed included women). I was astonished that the concept of not eating meat had never crossed my mind. I had never met a vegetarian nor heard of vegetarianism—this was 1962 America.

"One day my mother decided to cook a special treat. She bought some lobsters, filled the bathtub with water so they could await their fate in comfort, and put a big pot of water on to boil. As the live lobsters were dropped into the boiling water, I heard their screams. The thought crossed my mind, 'How could I cause such unspeakable suffering to my fellow beings, just because I liked the taste of their flesh?' I understood firsthand the yogic principle of ahimsa (non-violence) and never ate meat nor fish again."

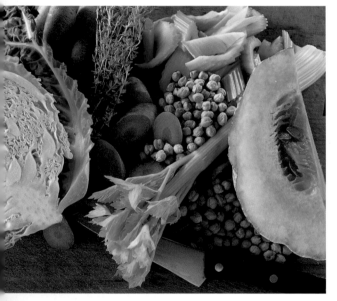

Swami Saradananda

The recipes in this book are in accord with the ancient philosophy of Yoga and Vedanta—the nondualistic philosophy that forms the metaphysical basis of yoga. Yoga prescribes a lactovegetarian diet for health and moral and spiritual reasons. This diet is an essential part of yoga, as it promotes a wellness that allows the rest of the discipline to proceed unhampered. A yogic diet is in itself a discipline of both body and mind, and is in accord with the spiritual principle of reverence for life, expressed as ahimsa.

"Purity of food brings purity of mind. Mind is the subtlest essence of food. An aspirant should be careful in the selection of articles of diet in the beginning of his spiritual life."

Swami Sivananda

Annamaya kosha (the physical body) is made of food. Our whole life can be seen as the effect of the interaction of food and life, or matter and energy, which are respectively food and the eater of food. Food is converted into energy, and energy uses food. Food is the door to a healthier life. It helps keep one free of bodily problems so the mind can concentrate and the spirit can grow. The process of cooking is a good discipline. It involves giving to others, organization, and frequently learning to work under pressure while staying calm. It also encourages cleanliness, imagination and responsibility. The yogic diet consists of pure vegetarian food freshly prepared with love. Perhaps as you achieve a proper, healthy diet you will be encouraged to tackle the other four principles of yoga—exercise; breathing; relaxation; and positive thinking and meditation. Even if you are interested only in the physical yoga exercises, you will be surprised by the enhancement of your practice as you modifiy your diet.

The Three Gunas

"Verily, this person consists of the essence of food."

Taittiriya Upanishad, II. 1

In yogic philosophy, the mind is formed from the subtlest portion or essence of food. If the food taken in is pure, the mind has the proper building materials for the development of a strong and subtle intellect and a good memory. A yogic diet brings inner peace to the body and mind and encourages spiritual progress.

All of Nature, including our diet, is catagorized into three qualities, or Gunas: sattvic (pure), rajasic (overstimulating), and tamasic (putrified). A person's mental makeup may be judged from the type of food he or she prefers to eat. Yogis believe not only that "you are what you eat," but also you eat those foods that reflect your own level of mental and spiritual purity. As your life changes in a positive way, you will also see your food preferences improving. The yogic diet is based on sattvic foods.

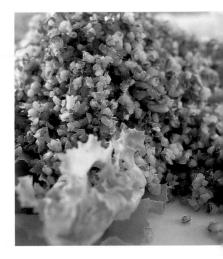

Sattvic Foods

"The foods which increase life, purity, strength, health, joy, and cheerfulness, which are savory and oleaginous, substantial and agreeable, are dear to the sattvic people."

Bhagavad Gita, XVII. 8

Pure foods that increase vitality, energy, vigor, health, and joy, that are delicious, wholesome, substantial, and agreeable are sattvic. These foods render the mind pure and calm and generate equanimity, poise and peaceful tendencies. Sattvic foods supply maximum energy, increase strength and endurance, and help to eliminate fatigue even for those who do strenuous work. They promote a peaceful attitude and are conducive to the practice of meditation.

Foods should be as fresh and natural as possible, preferably organically grown, not genetically modified, and kept without preservatives or artificial flavorings. They should also be eaten in as natural a state as possible—either raw, steamed, or cooked lightly.

Sattvic foods include:
Grains such as corn, barley, wheat, unpolished rice, oat, millet, and quinoa. Make sure you include in your diet coarse foods such as steel-cut oats and whole grain breads. These are good for the teeth and jaws, and they stimulate the processes of digestion and elimination. Grains supply necessary carbohydrates, the main source of energy for the body, and they also contain about half the amino acids (page 68) that are needed to form protein.

"Food makes thinking possible. Therefore the right food is of paramount importance. You must eat when you are in a cheerful mood. Do not overload the stomach."

Swami Sivananda

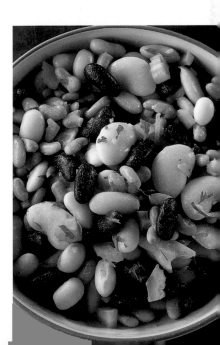

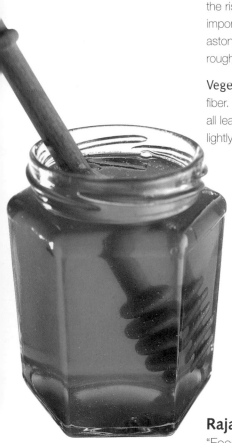

Protein foods such as legumes, nuts, and seeds. Proteins are the "building blocks" of the body. The key to a healthy vegetarian diet is to eat a good mixture of foods to make sure it includes all the amino acids essential for making proteins.

Fruits, both fresh and dried, as well as pure fruit juices, provided the ancient diet of the rishis and raja yogis. Among the many different foods, fruits stand foremost in importance in the yogis' menu or regime. The curative effects of fresh juicy fruits are astonishing. They fill the body with vitalizing, or life-giving, minerals and vitamins, and roughage (fiber). They contain alkaline matter that helps to keep the blood pure.

Vegetables are important in the diet because they contain minerals, vitamins, and fiber. The diet should include seeded vegetables (such as cucumbers and squashes), all leafy vegetables, and roots or tubers. These are best eaten raw or cooked as lightly as possible.

Herbs for seasoning and herbal teas.

Natural sweeteners, such as honey, molasses, maple syrup, and apple juice concentrate, are much better for you than processed sugar. Raw sugar is a traditional part of yogic diets in India, where, known as jaggery, it comes directly from the cane and is not processed. White sugar is best avoided in a healthy diet.

Dairy products, such as milk, butter, cheese, and yogurt, are traditionally an essential part of the yogic diet. However, modern dairy practices abuse the animals, filling their milk with hormones and antibiotics. We have, therefore, also suggested a vegan alternative for recipes, whenever possible. Even if you choose to use dairy products, we recommend you do so in moderation. They tend to intensify the production of mucus, which interferes with the natural flow of breath.

Rajasic Foods

"Foods that are bitter, sour, saline, excessively hot, pungent, dry, and burning, are liked by the Rajasic and are productive of pain, grief, and disease."

Bhagavad Gita, XVII. 9

The yogic diet avoids rajasic foods because they overstimulate the body and mind. They excite passions and boisterous tendencies, cause physical and mental stress, bring a restless state of mind, and destroy the mind-body balance that is essential for happiness. However, remember this division of foods into sattvic-rajasic-tamasic is a comparative one, not an absolute. It is meant to help you gain the insight to change your diet in a positive direction. Hence, spices are used in recipes, but they are used subtly and may be phased out as your tastes become "sattvic."

"The modern diet of fast food filled with chemicals and sugar has destroyed the body's natural balance. But yoga can help us to tune back into the body's true needs."

*Swami
Vishnu-devananda*

Onions, garlic, radishes, coffee, tea, tobacco, and stimulants of all kind fall into this category—also, heavily spiced and salted, chemical-riddled convenience foods and snacks. Sattvic food taken in the wrong place, such as "on the run," becomes rajasic. Refined (white) sugar, soft drinks, prepared mustards, pungent spices, highly seasoned foods, and anything excessively hot, bitter, sour, or saline are all rajasic and are best avoided.

Strong spices and condiments overstimulate the mind as well as irritate the mucus membrane of the intestines. Rajasic foods accentuate lust, anger, greed, selfishness, violence, and egoism, which are the barriers that separate people from each other and from their realization of the Divine. Rajas is the energy that creates dissension in life and wars in the world.

Tamasic Foods

"That food which is stale, tasteless, putrid, rotten, and impure refuse, is the food liked by the Tamasic."

Bhagavad Gita, XVII. 10

Tamasic food makes a person dull, inert, and lazy; it robs individuals of high ideals, purpose, and motivation. In addition, it accentuates the tendency to suffer from chronic ailments and depression, and fills the minds with darkness, anger, and impure thoughts. Abandoning tamasic foods needs to be among the first positive lifestyle changes you make.

Meat, fish, eggs, all intoxicants, alcoholic beverages, marijuana, and opium are tamasic in nature. Meat-eating and alcoholism are closely allied. The craving for alcohol dies a natural death when meat is withdrawn from the diet.

Tamasic foods include all foods that are stale, rotten, decomposed, unclean, as well as overripe and unripe fruits. Also included are foods that have been fermented, burned, fried, barbecued, or reheated many times: half-cooked, overcooked, and twice-cooked items, as well as stale products and those containing preservatives, for example canned, processed, and many prepared foods.

Mushrooms are included in this category, because they grow in the darkness. Also vinegar, because it is a product of fermentation and retards digestion.

Deep-fried foods are indigestible. The fat penetrates into them and the digestive juice of the stomach cannot act on them. The fine nutritive essence which is beneficial to health is destroyed by frying and the food takes on the quality of tamas.

Sattvic food taken in excessive quantity (overeating) becomes tamasic.

Guidelines for Healthy Eating

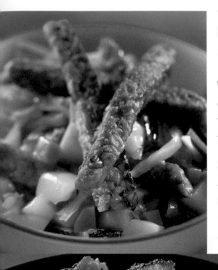

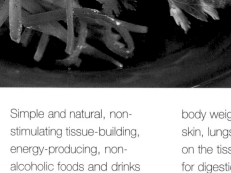

"From food all beings are born. Having been born, they grow by food. Food is eaten by all beings and it also eats them."

Taittiriya Upanishad, II. 2. 1

We go on in the circle of birth and death constantly. The body is born, grows, changes, decays, dies ... and is born again. Death means we now have to leave this physical body because of some karma (past action). This body came from food and goes back to the food chain.

Swami Vishnu-devananda illustrates this: "For example, I eat a nice red juicy tomato and my body grows. What happens to the tomato? It changes into my body. And my body itself is also constantly changing. One day it will die. Perhaps when you bury me you will put a tomato plant over the body. The tomato plant will say "You ate my cousin once upon a time. Now I'm going to eat you." Then beautiful tomatoes will grow. In this case, destruction of my body is construction of the tomato—and you all enjoy a nice tomato sauce!"

A diet which is not in agreement with the principles of satisfactory nutrition leads to impaired physical development, ill-health and untimely death. A high standard of health, vigor, and vitality can be achieved through a well-balanced diet. Such a diet will enable you to develop your inherited capacities to the full extent.

A well-balanced and adequate diet must yield enough calories, as well as supply the various food constituents in sufficient quantities. We need both an energy source for our day-to-day functioning, and vitamins and minerals to stimulate the production of particular hormones and to prevent debilitative diseases.

Simple and natural, non-stimulating tissue-building, energy-producing, non-alcoholic foods and drinks keep the mind calm and pure, and help the yogic practitioner to attain the goal of life.

Water is also a necessary part of the diet. About 70 percent of the body weight is water. There is a daily loss of about $1\frac{1}{2}$ quarts of water through the skin, lungs, kidneys, and the alimentary canal. Water has a greater cleansing action on the tissues than other beverages. It dissolves and distributes food. It is necessary for digestion, and removes impurities from the body. It keeps the body temperature equable through evaporation from the skin in the form of sweat.

Make all changes in your diet gradually. If something disagrees with you, reduce the quantity or eliminate it completely. With practice, you will develop an inner voice to guide you in the selection of a diet suited to your temperament and constitution; one that will maintain your physical efficiency, good health, and mental vigor.

Life may be a continual battle, but it is also a never-ending adventure. There are many dragons to be destroyed. You will have to wage war with the enemies of health—impure water, bad ventilation, overwork, unwholesome food, disease germs, domestic pests such as mosquitos and flies. We are surrounded on all sides by invisible foes, the pathogenic or disease-causing microbes or bacteria. You should learn all you can about your enemies—their ways, habits, and strengths. However, you can also fortify yourself by developing your inner strengths, following these healthy eating guidelines:

● Always respect your food. Begin each meal by giving thanks for it.

● Maintain a peaceful attitude during meals; observe silence if you are alone. When eating with family and friends, try not to argue or discuss unpleasant experiences. Genial conversation can create the balanced, loving environment that enhances digestion and amplifies the body's ability to assimilate the food's nourishment.

● Do not eat when you are angry. Rest for a while until your mind becomes calm and then take some food. Poisons are secreted by the glands and thrown into the bloodstream when you are angry and upset.

● Do not eat food that is too hot, nor too cold, because this will upset the stomach and produce indigestion.

● Do not force yourself to eat anything you do not like, but also do not eat only those foods you like the most.

● Abandon too many mixtures or combinations of foods. They are difficult for the system to digest. Eat moderately what you find agreeable. A simple diet is best.

● Eat at least one raw dish in each meal to keep your blood alkaline.

● Try to refrain from drinking during a meal as this will dilute the gastric juice, causing indigestion and other stomach complaints.

● Keep the mouth sweet and clean—it is the gatekeeper of the digestive system.

● Eat slowly and savor your food. Chew it thoroughly, remembering that digestion of food begins in the mouth. Appetizing food and thorough chewing stimulate the flow of saliva and other digestive juices.

● Eat moderately. The secret of being healthy and happy is always to be a little hungry. Don't overload the stomach. Overeating hinders elimination, assimilation, and growth, making the organs overworked, stressed, and vulnerable to disease.

● Gluttons and epicureans cannot even dream of succeeding in yoga. Whoever regulates their diet can become a yogi. Take half a stomachful of food, a quarter stomachful of water, and allow the remaining quarter free for the expansion of gas.

Simple, wholesome, pure foods help to neutralize waste material and poisons, and cleanse the system thoroughly.

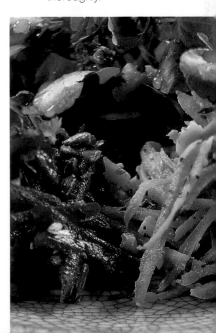

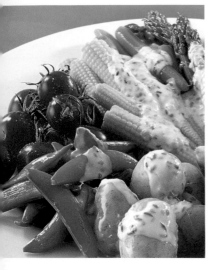

• Eat at fixed times; try to refrain from eating between meals. If you do not feel hungry at mealtime, fast until the next meal. Eat only when you are really hungry. Beware of false hunger. The gastric fire is God. Wait for the appearance of this God within and only then offer Him some food.

• Try to eat as little processed food as possible.

• Foods are best when cooked lightly. Overcooking robs them of their nutritional value and flavor.

• Try not to eat large meals late at night. Do not eat rice or beans at this time, because they are heavy to digest and you will find it difficult to get up for meditation in the morning. If you are very hungry, eat something light—perhaps fruit.

• Eat to live, don't live to eat. You need food to maintain body heat, produce new cells, and repair wear and tear. Be simple in your eating habits. The person who practices regular meditation wants very little food.

• Take some lemon and honey in the morning for health and energy, and to purify the blood.

"Moderate diet is defined to mean taking pleasant and sweet food, leaving one-fourth of the stomach free, and offering the act up to the Lord."

Hatha Yoga Pradipika, I. 58

• Do not practice asanas immediately after eating, nor when you are hungry. Also, it is not advisable to do any strenuous physical or mental work immediately after eating. In the morning, when physical and nervous forces are at their most vigorous, the stomach can proceed with its functions if the breakfast is followed by moderate exercise, such as a leisurely walk to the bus. After supper there should not be any work, but recreation. This is when bodily vigor is at its lowest and should not be taxed farther.

• Try sitting in Vajra Asana (sitting on the heels with knees and feet together) for 10 minutes after a meal; this will assist digestion.

• Do not become a slave to food and drink. Do not make much fuss about diet. Take simple and natural foods. If you think too much about food this will create more body-consciousness.

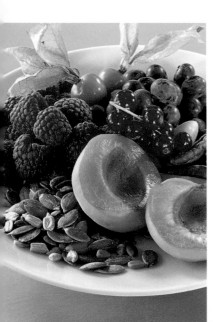

• Try fasting one day per week. Fasting eliminates poisons, overhauls the internal mechanism, and gives rest to the organs.

• Remember God, the indweller of all foods, the bestower of all bounties. Remember God during meals and give thanks to God just before and after eating.

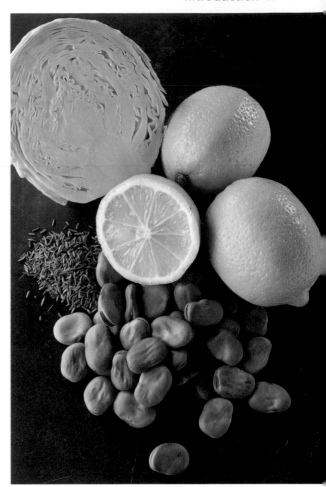

"We are constantly bombarded with stimuli, and these make up the diet of our lifestyle. From the food we eat, the air we breath, the things we see, feel, hear, and touch our environment is formed, and this, in turn, profoundly influences and shapes our internal environment. We are what we eat—literally, for the mind is constructed out of the sublest parts of our diet and the body from the rest. To achieve the goal of life, to find contentment and perfection requires a peaceful and focused mind. To control the mind is difficult since it is in reality very much under the control of our physical body. It is therefore suggested we first dis- cipline and control the physical body and then the mind may be easily controlled. Diet plays an important part in this process."

Swami Vishnu-devananda

Replacement Foods

The following are substitutions you can make in standard recipes to help you to make a gradual change to a yogic diet.

Food	Yogic replacement
Cheese, grated	Yeast flakes
Cottage cheese	Tofu, crumbled
Eggs—as binder	1 tablespoon peanut butter, tahini, or blended tofu per egg, or 1 teaspoon soy flour
Eggs—as leavening agent	Baking powder or yogurt plus sparkling mineral water
Eggs—as protein source	Tofu (plus a pinch of turmeric, if desired)
Flesh foods	Tofu, tempeh, legumes (beans)
Milk	Soy milk, nut and seed milks, oat milk, rice milk
Onions	Cabbage, celery or turnips
Vinegar	Lemon juice

Making Positive Changes in Your Life

Eating a wholesome diet is a good start to making positive changes; it is the opening of a door to a healthier and happier way of life. Some changes may seem easy, but others take a bit longer. The following suggestions, combined with yoga exercises, will help you make the positive changes permanent ones. Yoga sessions begin with a few minutes relaxation in the Corpse pose. The asanas begin with the Sun Salutation, a warming-up exercise. OM is the original mantra, the root of all sounds and letters (see Glossary, page 156).

	1 to 7 weeks	2 to 6 months	6 months to 1 year	2 to 3 years	Continuing on
Proper exercise	12 Basic asanas + Sun Salutation.	Add simple variations.	Add Intermediate variations.	Intermediate/ Advanced asanas.	Advanced asanas.
Proper breathing	Practice deep abdominal breathing.	Learn basic pranayama.	Practice 15 to 30 min. pranayama daily.	Practice 30 min. pranayama daily.	Practice 30 to 45 min. pranayama daily.
Proper relaxation	Learn Corpse pose.	Relax in Corpse pose 15 min. daily.	Relax in Corpse pose 15 min. daily.	Relax in Corpse pose 15 min. daily.	Relax in Corpse pose 15 min. daily.
Reduce negative dietary habits	Eliminate meat and fish from your diet. Cut down on fried foods.	Eliminate eggs from your diet. Cut down on soft drinks and candy.	Cut down on heavily salted and convenience foods.	Eliminate stale, burned, and tamasic foods.	Eliminate onions, garlic, and other rajasic foods from your diet.
Reinforcing positive dietary habits	Drink 4 to 5 glasses of water and eat one raw salad daily.	Increase intake of legumes and tofu.	Eat food as freshly prepared as possible.	Eat at least one meal per week in silence.	Practice thankfulness at each meal.
Fasting	Replace one meal each week with a glass of freshly made juice.	Fast on water or fresh juices for one day each week.	Once a year, do a 3-day fast on water or fresh juices. Practice kriyas.	Once or twice a year, do a 3-day fast on water or fresh juices.	Fast twice a year: once, for a week, on vegetable juices; for the other, do 3 days on water.
Eradicating negative habits	If you use marijuana or any other drugs, replace them with abdominal breathing.	Stop smoking. If you want a cigarette, do breathing exercises.	Cut down and eventually eliminate the intake of alcohol.	Begin to cut down on consumption of of coffee, tea, and other stimulants.	Evaluate your bad habits and try to eliminate them, one by one.
Concentration exercises	Let go of the past and future, focusing only in the present.	Practice listening and hearing what others are saying.	Practice Tratak (candle gazing exercise) daily.	Mentally repeat OM, or other mantra, 10 min. daily.	Practice focusing on one thing at a time.
Positive thinking	Refrain from using abusive language.	Try to spend time with people who have a positive outlook on life.	Stop procrastinating. Put positive ideas into practice as soon as possible.	Remove words like "can't" from your vocabulary (including your mental vocabulary).	Begin to see your failures as stepping stones to success; view as learning experiences.
Meditation	Sit silently for at least 20 minutes daily with the mind focused on breath.	Mentally repeat a mantra, such as OM, tuning it to the breath.	Increase your time of sitting to 30 min. daily.	With regular practice, the mind becomes less jumpy.	Continue the regular practice and you will experience peace.
Study	Read something of inspiration daily.	Study some verses of scripture or poetry that are uplifting.	Develop a contemplative attitude by seeing how these verses apply to your life.	Attend discourses or workshops that discuss inspirational readings.	Continue to study daily, trying to put your learnings into practice in your daily life.

A Prayer Before Meals

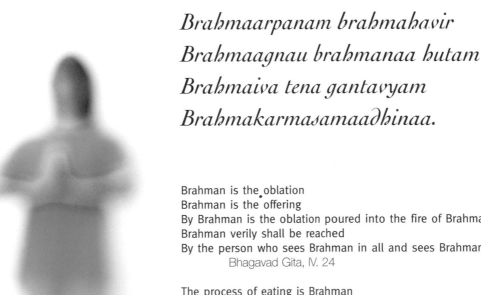

ब्रह्मार्पणं ब्रह्महविर्ब्रह्माग्नौ ब्रह्मणा हुतम् ।
ब्रह्मैव तेन गन्तव्यं ब्रह्मकर्मसमाधिना ॥ २४ ॥

Brahmaarpanam brahmahavir
Brahmaagnau brahmanaa hutam
Brahmaiva tena gantavyam
Brahmakarmasamaadhinaa.

Brahman is the oblation
Brahman is the offering
By Brahman is the oblation poured into the fire of Brahman
Brahman verily shall be reached
By the person who sees Brahman in all and sees Brahman in all action.
Bhagavad Gita, IV. 24

The process of eating is Brahman
The offering (the food itself) is Brahman
The person (the eater) who is doing the offering (the eating) is Brahman,
and the (gastric) fire by which the food is consumed is also Brahman
Thus by seeing Brahman everywhere in action, one reaches that Divine State
(Brahman).

YOGIC START
TO THE DAY

"Be sober and temperate; you will be healthy. Bask in the sun; spend time in the open air. The sun and the open air are your good doctor. Let your food be simple. Never eat too much, but don't eat too little. Take sufficient exercise. Become your own physician."

Swami Sivananda

A much-neglected meal, breakfast all too often consists of a quick bowl of boxed cereal and hasty cup(s) of coffee. As most nutritionists emphasize this is the most important meal of the day, we include a range of healthy recipes that can be prepared with a minimum of fuss, to set you up for the day.

Breakfast can be a light or more substantial meal depending on your eating patterns, but it is best not to miss it. Eating a healthy breakfast makes it less likely that you will capitulate to unhealthy, midmorning snacks or be so ravenous by lunchtime that you overeat. Children, in particular, need a good breakfast, otherwise they tend to become listless and have difficulty concentrating.

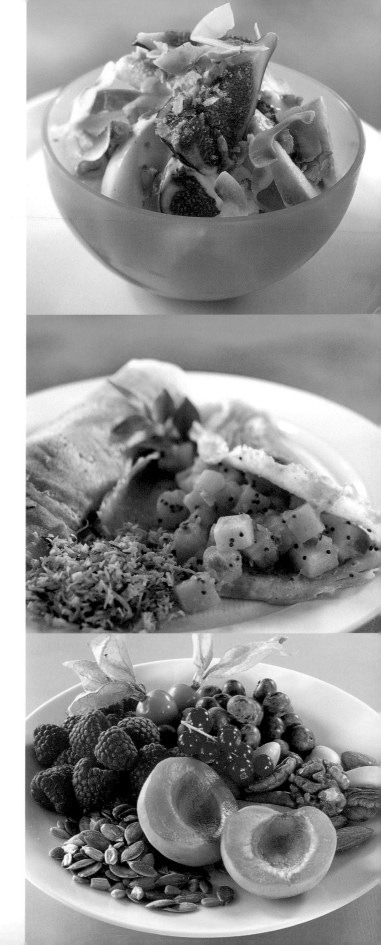

In Sivananda ashrams (monasteries or quiet places where one practices yoga) around the world the daily routine includes two substantial meals, to fit in with the program of asanas and meditation. Breakfast is eaten at 10 a.m., after morning meditation and asanas. Usually everyone is ready for a substantial meal by this time, especially as the next meal is not served until 6 p.m.

The morning meal, more than any other, reminds us of the essential function of food—to fuel our bodies. When most of us think of breakfast, only a few foods and beverages come to mind. But here we offer an interesting and health-filled variety to choose from. As with all meals, the good breakfast should strike a balance between the different categories of food. Whole grains, in the form of cereals, breads, or pancakes, provide a rich source of complex carbohydrates. The inclusion of fruits satisfies the longing for sweetness. Protein in the form of tofu or legumes helps to raise the basal metabolic rate, giving a feeling of energy and well-being.

Ginger-Carrot Juice

Starting with natural raw foods gives you stamina and energy to cope with the stress and strains of the day. Carrots are a good tonic for the brain, rich in vitamin A and minerals such as calcium. As well as nourishing the body in general, this juice will clear the lungs. The warming properties of ginger improve circulation and help the prana to flow freely. This is wonderful when you are on a juice fast. The apples or celery in this recipe can be omitted, if preferred, and you can vary the amount of ginger according to personal taste. About 3 cups roughly chopped cabbage may be substituted for the apples. Use organic carrots and apples, if possible; if they are not organic, peel them. Serves 4

2 crisp, juicy eating apples, quartered
3 carrots, scrubbed
1 stick of celery

½-to 1-inch piece of fresh gingerroot, peeled, or a pinch of ground ginger
¾ cup plus 2 tablespoons water
Juice of ½ lemon or 1 whole lime

1 If you have a juicer, use it to juice the apples, carrots, celery, and piece of gingerroot. Alternatively, chop the carrots and celery, place in a food processor with the apples and ginger, and process to a pulp, then press out the juice through a fine strainer.

2 Dilute the juice with the water. Stir in the lemon or lime juice and the ground ginger, if using. Serve at once.

Minty Tomato Juice

A refreshing and cleansing early-morning drink. Tomatoes, however, are too acidic to use while fasting. The combined warming effect of the tomato, lime, and cayenne pepper makes this a wonderful tonic for winter. Fresh juices are the most vital and regenerating of foods, containing readily available energy to nourish the cells of the body. Serves 4 to 6

4½ cups tomato juice
3 tablespoons fresh lime juice
2 tablespoons finely chopped fresh mint

Pinch of cayenne pepper (optional)
Lime slices, to garnish

Combine the tomato juice, lime juice, mint, and cayenne pepper, if using. Pour into individual glasses and serve as soon as possible, garnished with lime slices.

Almond Milk
This sustaining and soothing drink was developed by Swami Vishnu-devananda during the time he was doing intensive sadhana (yogic practice) in the Himalayas. It is served daily during the Sivananda Sadhana intensive courses which are run for yoga teachers, as it is a rich source of easily digestible food for the rapid replenishment of energy. Almonds are a concentrated source of protein, as well as being high in vitamins and minerals such as iron, magnesium, potassium, and zinc. Their fat content makes them excellent for skin and muscle repair. Highly valued in Ayurveda (the traditional Indian medical system), almonds strengthen the respiratory system and lubricate the intestines. The ingredients below are per person; simply multiply them by the number of people you want to serve. Recipe per person

10 almonds, soaked overnight in enough
  water to cover
Pinch of ground cardamom

Pinch of pepper
1 cup warm milk, water, or soy milk
1 teaspoon honey

1 Drain the almonds, reserving the soaking water, and remove the skins. Place the nuts in a food processor or blender with the soaking water and the cardamom and pepper. Blend at high speed for 5 minutes.

2 Combine the almond mixture with the warm milk, water, or soy milk. Stir in the honey. Drink at once.

Citrus Slices with Pomegranate Seeds
An attractive fruit salad such as this one is the perfect way to brighten a gray morning! The pomegranate seeds invigorate the system while cooling and strengthening it, and they are an excellent blood purifier. The ginger gives the salad some bite, as well as stimulating digestion. Serves 4 to 6

1 orange
1 pink grapefruit
1 or 2 kiwi fruit (optional)

½ pomegranate
1 tablespoon finely chopped crystallized
  ginger (optional)

1 Peel the citrus fruit and slice into ¼-inch thick slices, or divide into segments, removing as much pith as possible. Slice or quarter the kiwi fruit, if using.

2 Arrange the fruit on a serving platter. Scoop out the pomegranate seeds with a spoon, omitting the pulp around them. Sprinkle the pomegranate seeds and chopped crystallized ginger, if using, over the top of the fruit. Serve at once.

- If pomegranate seeds are not available, use black grapes to add color to this dish.
- Substitute chopped fresh mint leaves for the crystallized ginger.
- Fresh, sliced pineapple is also a welcome ingredient.

Apple-Fig Salad Serves 6

6 dried or fresh figs
2 eating apples and 2 bananas, sliced
1¾ cups chopped walnuts
2 tablespoons unsweetened dried coconut

1 tablespoon lemon juice
4 tablespoons honey
½ cup plain yogurt, sour cream, or Toasted
   Nut Dream (page 115) (optional)

If using dried figs, soak them in cold water for 1 to 2 hours, then drain. Cut the fresh or dried figs into quarters. Stir the fruit, nuts, coconut, lemon juice, and honey together. Serve at once, topped with yogurt, sour cream, or toasted nut dream, if desired.

Baked Bananas *There is an old Indian folk saying: "Bananas are gold in the morning, silver at noon, and lead at night." Their high carbohydrate content makes them the perfect breakfast food for an active lifestyle, and their potassium content encourages muscle pliancy—if you suffer from muscle cramps, bananas will help to alleviate them. The students at our yoga centers and ashrams consume vast amounts of the fruit for this reason.* Serves 4 to 8

4 bananas
⅓ cup maple syrup
½ cup orange juice
⅓ cup chopped or slivered almonds

¼ teaspoon ground cardamom
4 tablespoons butter or margarine, melted
Grated fresh coconut or toasted, unsweetened
   dried coconut for sprinkling (optional)

1 Heat the oven to 400°F. Peel the bananas and halve them lengthwise. Lay them in a baking dish.

2 Combine the maple syrup, orange juice, almonds, cardamom, and melted butter or margarine. Pour the mixture over the bananas and bake in the oven for 30 minutes. Serve at once, topped with grated or toasted dried coconut, if desired.

Winter Compote Serves 4 to 6

7 ounces dried apricots
4 ounces prunes
4 ounces dried pears
4 ounces dried apples

6 cloves
1 cinnamon stick
1 tablespoon apple juice concentrate
2½ cups water

1 Place the dried fruit in a bowl with the spices, apple juice concentrate, and water and leave to soak overnight.

2 The next morning, transfer the mixture to a pan and bring to a boil. Reduce the heat, half cover the pan, and simmer for 25 minutes, stirring occasionally. Remove the spices and serve.

• Winter Fruit Shake: If you don't have time to prepare the compote, you can make it into this quick shake, which combines the nourishment of dried fruits with protein-rich soy milk for a wonderful morning energy booster. Omit the cloves, cinnamon stick, apple juice concentrate, and water. Place the dried fruits (it doesn't matter if they are soaked or not) in a food processor or blender with 1 to 2¼ cups soy milk (or milk, if preferred). Add ½ teaspoon ground cinnamon, if desired. Blend until smooth and serve.

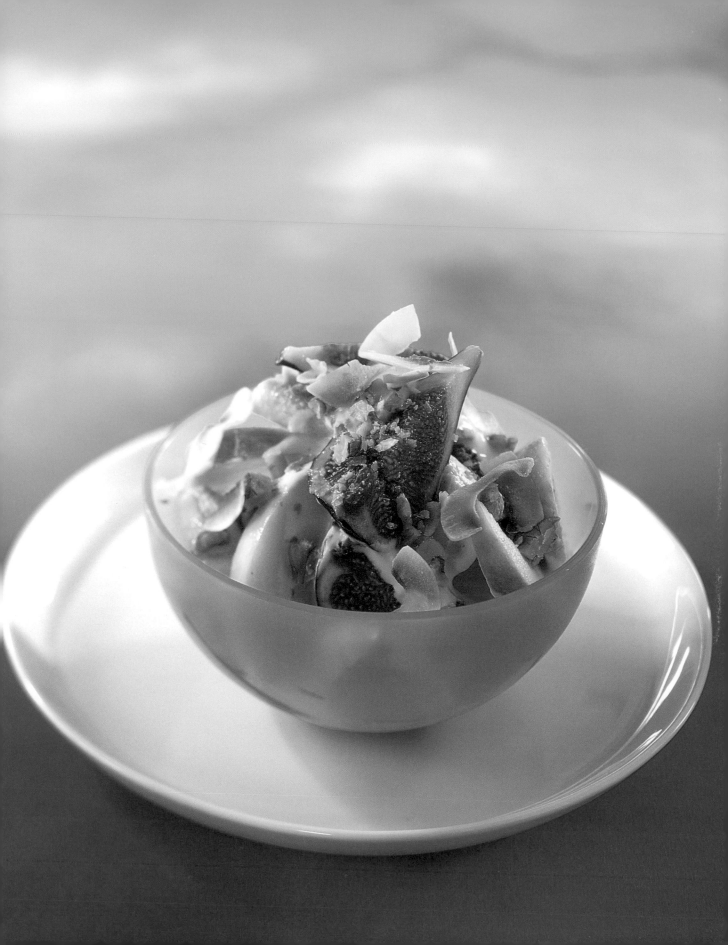

Granola

There are many recipes for granola. This one does not contain any added oil, but includes a wonderful array of grains, nuts, and seeds—a veritable treasure-house of natural oils, minerals, and vitamins! At our Yoga Retreat on Paradise Island, Bahamas, we pick fresh coconuts off the trees. When opened, the coconut pulp is shredded and ⅔ cup (unpacked) is toasted along with the grain mixture. Sweetened dried coconut can be used as a variation. If adding coconut, the liquid sweetener can be reduced. You can simplify the recipe by increasing the quantities of some ingredients if you do not have others. Granola can be made in advance and stored in an airtight container in a cool place (not the refrigerator) for several weeks. To serve, simply add some milk, yogurt, or soy milk. Makes 12 to 16 servings

½ cup maple syrup
½ cup hot water
½ teaspoon vanilla extract
3¾ cups rolled oats
5 cups rye, millet, or wheat flakes
8½ tablespoons wheat germ or bran

¾ cup hazelnuts, almonds, or any other nuts
1 cup sunflower seeds
⅓ cup sesame seeds
½ cup golden raisins or raisins
⅓ cup chopped dates or other dried
    fruits (optional)

1 Heat the oven to 250°F. Combine the maple syrup, hot water, and vanilla extract.

2 Mix the grains, nuts, and seeds in a large mixing bowl. Stir in the maple syrup and vanilla solution and mix thoroughly. Spread out the mixture on a lightly greased baking sheet and bake in the oven for about 1 hour, stirring three or four times to prevent it from burning. The granola is ready when it is lightly brown.

3 Mix the granola with the dried fruit while still warm, breaking up the larger chunks as you do so. Leave to cool and then store in airtight containers.

Oatmeal-Yogurt Cream

The Sivananda Yoga International Headquarters is in maple syrup-producing Quebec, Canada, so we always have supplies on hand. However, if you don't have ready access, you can use barley malt syrup, rice syrup, date syrup, or honey. Serves 3 to 4

⅓ cup finely chopped almonds
½ cup rolled oats
Grated zest and juice of ½ lemon or orange

2 tablespoons maple syrup, or sweetener of
    choice
1¼ cups creamy plain yogurt
1 tablespoon chopped almonds, toasted

1 Heat the broiler. Mix together the chopped almonds and oats. Spread out on a baking sheet and place under the hot broiler for about 2 minutes, stirring frequently to brown evenly. Leave to cool.

2 Mix the lemon or orange zest and juice with the sweetener and stir into the yogurt. Fold in the almond mixture. Spoon into individual glass dishes and chill until required.

3 Top with toasted chopped almonds and serve at once.

Apple Muesli
A quick-and-easy recipe for when time is short. Oats are renowned for their energy-giving properties, as well as the warmth they give to the body. Because they are very alkaline, they relieve tension and help you to practice "proper relaxation." Serves 4 to 6

⅓ cup raisins
⅔ cup unsweetened apple juice
2 eating apples, cored and coarsely chopped
Generous 3 cups rolled oats

1 tablespoon honey
2 tablespoons slivered almonds
Milk, yogurt, or soy milk, to serve

1 Soak the raisins in the apple juice for 20 minutes. Put the chopped apples into a bowl, add the raisins and apple juice and toss to combine them.

2 Stir in the rolled oats and honey. Add the almonds and stir well to mix everything together. Serve at once with milk, yogurt, or soy milk.

• Double the amount of the apple juice; soak the raisins and oatmeal overnight. Add the other ingredients in the morning.

Orange Couscous
For a refreshingly different start to the day, try this dish instead of oatmeal. In summer, fresh apricots or peaches can be used. The toasted coconut provides a rich texture to the dish, which can be served plain or with yogurt, milk, or soy milk. Serves 4 to 6

12 dried apricots, thinly sliced
2¼ cups orange juice
¼ teaspoon salt
1 cup couscous

3 tablespoons grated fresh or unsweetened dried coconut, toasted
1 orange, peeled and divided into segments, to serve (optional)

1 Place the apricots, orange juice, and salt in a saucepan and bring to a boil. Stir in the couscous and remove from the heat. Cover the pan and let it stand for 5 minutes, until the liquid is absorbed by the couscous; the couscous should be light and fluffy, but still slightly grainy to the bite.

2 Place in individual serving bowls. Top each portion with a little toasted coconut and orange segments, if desired. Serve warm.

• **Apple-Cinnamon Bulgur:** Put 2 roughly chopped crisp eating apples, 2¼ cups unsweetened apple juice, ⅓ cup raisins or golden raisins, ¼ teaspoon ground cinnamon, and ¼ teaspoon salt into a saucepan and bring to a boil. Stir in 1¼ cups bulgur wheat. Cover and simmer over low heat for about 15 minutes, until all the liquid is absorbed. Serve warm, sprinkled with chopped nuts or sunflower seeds.

Uppama with Mixed Vegetables *A South Indian*
breakfast or supper dish. Serve with Coconut Chutney (page 125) or yogurt. Serves 6

3½ cups coarse semolina
2 cups diced potatoes
¾ teaspoon paprika and ¾ teaspoon turmeric
Salt
½ cup oil
1½ teaspoons black mustard seeds
1½ teaspoons cumin seeds
3 tomatoes, chopped

1½-inch piece fresh gingerroot, peeled and finely chopped
3 fresh green chilies, seeded and finely chopped (optional)
10 ounces mixed vegetables (carrots, cabbage, green bell pepper), very finely chopped or grated
3⅓ cups boiling water
A few sprigs of fresh cilantro leaves, chopped

1 Heat a large skillet or wok. Add the semolina and cook over low heat for 10 to 12 minutes, until it is a few shades darker, stirring constantly. Remove from the pan; set aside.

2 Sprinkle the potatoes with paprika, turmeric, and a little salt. Heat the oil in the skillet. Add the potatoes and sauté over medium heat until brown. Remove with a slotted spoon; set aside.

3 Add the mustard and cumin seeds to the skillet and heat them over high heat until they begin to "pop." Add the tomatoes, ginger, and chilies, if using, and stir well over low heat. Add the mixed vegetables and cook for 5 minutes.

4 Add the boiling water and 1 teaspoon salt. Gradually add the toasted semolina, stirring all the time; the mixture should be light and crumbly without any lumps. Add a little more water if the mixture is too dry. Gently mix in the fried potatoes, and garnish with cilantro leaves. Serve at once.

Dosas *These light crepes are a typical breakfast in South India. The rice and urid dal (a type of white lentil available from Indian food stores) combine to make perfectly balanced protein. Serve with Coconut Chutney (page 125) and Sambar (page 140). Or stuff with Curried Potato (page 88) to make Masala Dosa.* Serves 4 to 6

¾ cup urid dal, washed
1½ cups basmati rice
3½ cups water

1 teaspoon crushed fenugreek (optional)
1 teaspoon salt
Ghee or oil for cooking

1 Place the urid dal and rice in separate bowls. Add 1¼ cups of the water to the urid dal and stir in the fenugreek, if using. Add the rest of the water to the rice. Leave to soak for at least 12 hours, then grind them separately in a food processor or blender with the water they have been soaked in, grinding until smooth, adding a little more water if necessary. Combine the urid dal and rice to make a runny batter. Leave to stand in a warm place for 8 hours, or overnight—it will get slightly thicker and fizzy.

2 Heat a heavy skillet or griddle over medium heat and grease very lightly with greased paper towel. Stir the salt into the batter, which should be a thick, pouring consistency. Drop a ladleful of batter (about 3 tablespoons) into the pan. Using the back of the ladle, very gently swirl the batter from the center outward to make a thin, crepelike dosa.

3 Cook over medium heat until the edges of the dosa start to lift, 1 to 3 minutes. Brush very lightly with ghee or oil and turn it over—if you try and turn it over too soon before it has started to set, the dosa will break. Cook until golden brown. Serve at once.

Dosas with Curried Potato and Coconut Chutney

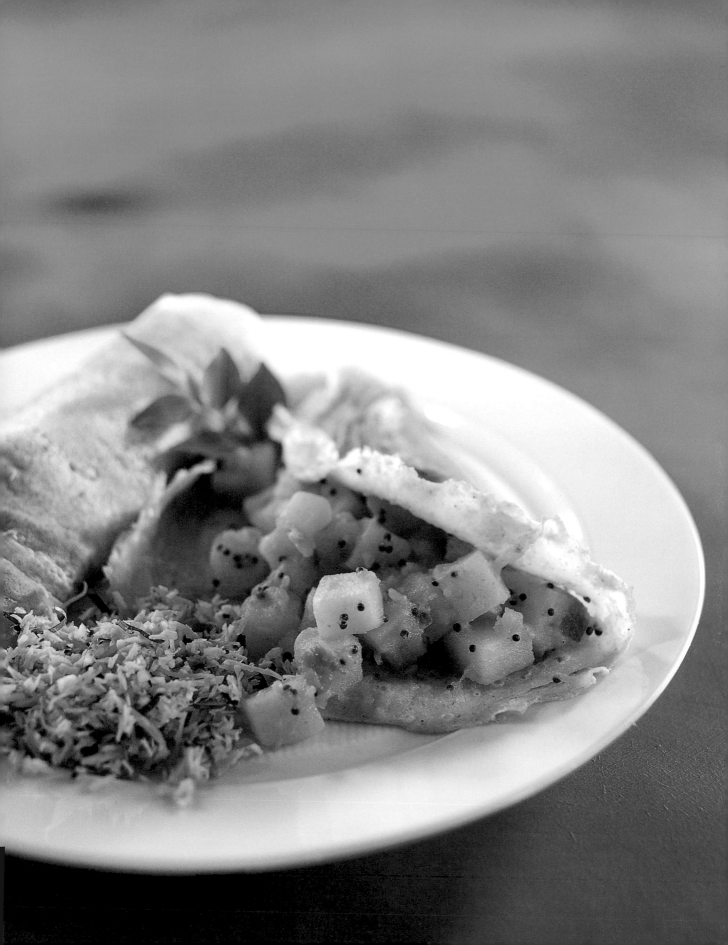

Wheat-Free Crepes
For breakfast or a snack, these light, crispy crepes are so good they can be served plain or with maple syrup. For a festive breakfast, serve them hot with Baked Bananas (page 24). They can also be filled with either a sweet or savory filling, folded, and topped with syrup or a sauce. Serves 4 to 6

1½ cups stirred soy flour
1¾ cups rice flour
1 tablespoon baking powder
Pinch of salt
1½ cups water

1 to 2 teaspoons honey
4 tablespoons oil
Oil for frying
Maple syrup or Raisin Sauce (page 114), to serve

1 Combine the soy flour, rice flour, baking powder, and salt. Add the water a little at a time, stirring so the batter is smooth. Gradually beat in the honey and the oil—the batter should be very runny.

2 Heat a heavy skillet over high heat. Reduce the heat to medium and brush with oil. Add a ladleful of batter to the pan and flatten out thinly with the back of a spoon. Fry until the center bubbles, turn it over, and cook until golden brown. Repeat with the remaining batter to make 10 to 12 crepes. Serve hot, with maple syrup or raisin sauce.

• **Buckwheat Pancakes:** This traditional American favorite is frequently served on Sunday morning at our Catskill Mountain Yoga Ranch in New York. Combine 1¼ cups whole wheat flour, ¾ cup buckwheat flour, ⅓ cup powdered milk, and 1 teaspoon baking powder in a mixing bowl. Gradually add enough water to make a runny consistency, then beat in 4 tablespoons molasses, 2 tablespoons plain yogurt, and 2 tablespoons oil. Cook spoonfuls of the batter to make chunkier pancakes, 4 to 5 inches in diameter. Cook three or four at a time. As each pancake is removed from the pan, top with a pat of butter and place the next pancake on top, repeating the layers to make a stack of four to six pancakes per person. Pour maple syrup or Raisin Sauce (page 114) made with a little extra water over each stack. Each person gets a stack. To eat, the stacks are sliced like a cake and eaten slice by slice, rather than pancake by pancake.

Fruit Toast
An interesting departure from the more traditional cinnamon toast. This recipe needs a little preparation, but is a wonderfully satisfying weekend breakfast. Any seasonal fruit may be used. Recipe per person

1 teaspoon butter or margarine
1 peach, nectarine, or apple, or 2 apricots, sliced
2 teaspoons sugar-free whole fruit apricot or peach jam

1 teaspoon lemon juice (optional)
1 slice light rye or sunflower seed bread, lightly toasted

1 Heat the oven to 400°F. Melt the butter or margarine in a large, heavy-based saucepan or skillet and sauté the fruit for 2 to 3 minutes, until it begins to soften. Turn off the heat and stir in the fruit jam and lemon juice, if using.

2 Place the toast on a baking sheet and spoon the fruit mixture on top of it. Bake in the oven for 5 to 10 minutes. Serve immediately.

Carrot and Molasses Muffins

Special thanks go to Martha and to Swami Premananda for these recipes. Muffins should come out of the oven nicely golden with a moist center. Problems are usually caused by the batter being too dry or too wet; if necessary, add more water, oil, or flour to bring it to a wet and sticky consistency (not runny), but take care not to overmix the ingredients or the muffins will be heavy; the correct consistency is like mud. For richer muffins, replace some of the water with milk or soy milk. Buttermilk is especially good, as it helps the muffins to rise. These muffins are made with finely ground whole wheat flour called whole wheat pastry flour, available from health-food stores. Makes 12 large muffins

2¼ cups finely grated raw carrots or
   3 cups mashed, cooked carrots
4 cups unsifted whole wheat pastry flour
1½ cups stirred soy flour
1 teaspoon ground cinnamon

2¼ cups chopped dates
1⅓ cups chopped nuts (optional)
⅓ cup molasses
¾ cup oil
4 tablespoons water

1 Heat the oven to 350°F. Combine the raw or cooked carrots, flours, cinnamon, dates, and nuts, if using. Mix the molasses, oil, and water in a separate large bowl.

2 Add the molasses and oil mixture to the carrot mixture and fold together quickly until all the dry ingredients are moistened and evenly mixed.

3 Spoon into greased muffin pans and bake in the oven for 20 to 30 minutes, until a fine skewer or fork inserted into the center of a muffin comes out clean. Serve at once.

Savory Cheese Muffins

Makes 12 large muffins

1¾ cups grated vegetarian cheese
2 teaspoons dried oregano
5 cups whole wheat flour
1 cup grated carrots
¾ cup finely chopped zucchini, or ⅔ cup cored,
   seeded, and finely chopped green bell pepper

Scant ½ cup canned corn kernels
1 teaspoon dried basil
1 tablespoon baking powder
1 teaspoon salt and ¼ teaspoon pepper
2¼ cups soy milk or buttermilk
1 cup oil

1 Heat the oven to 350°F. Set aside a scant ½ cup of the grated cheese and 1 teaspoon of the oregano. Combine all the rest of the ingredients, except the soy milk or buttermilk and oil, in a bowl. In a separate large bowl, mix the milk and oil together.

2 Add the milk and oil mixture to the dry mixture and fold together quickly until the dry ingredients are moistened and evenly mixed.

3 Spoon into greased muffin pans. Mix the reserved cheese and oregano together and sprinkle it over the top of the muffins. Bake in the oven for 20 to 30 minutes, until a fine skewer or fork inserted into the center of a muffin comes out clean. Serve at once.

- For a vegan version, use soy cheese.
- For a wheat-free version, replace the wheat flour with buckwheat or spelt flour.
- Substitute yellow cornmeal for half the whole wheat flour.
- Use other fresh or dried herb combinations of your choice.

SOUP
SAMSKARAS

*"Eat moderately what you know
by experience is agreeable to
you and what is digestible.
Simple diet is best."*

Swami Sivananda

"Samskaras" are the subtle impressions formed in the conscious and subconscious minds by our daily activities and experiences. When the body is properly nourished, samskaras of strength are imprinted and we feel better able to deal with the stresses of life.

For the start of a meal, or as a main meal in itself, soups are nutritious, satisfying, and easy to prepare. Nothing is more warming or fulfilling than a hearty bowl of soup on a cold day—it nourishes both body and soul. On a warm summer's day, a refreshing light soup rejuvenates the mind and invigorates the prana. Soups can be an innovative and economical way to feed a family or group of friends using simple ingredients and techniques. Soups can also be an easy, yet substantial, meal for people with busy lives.

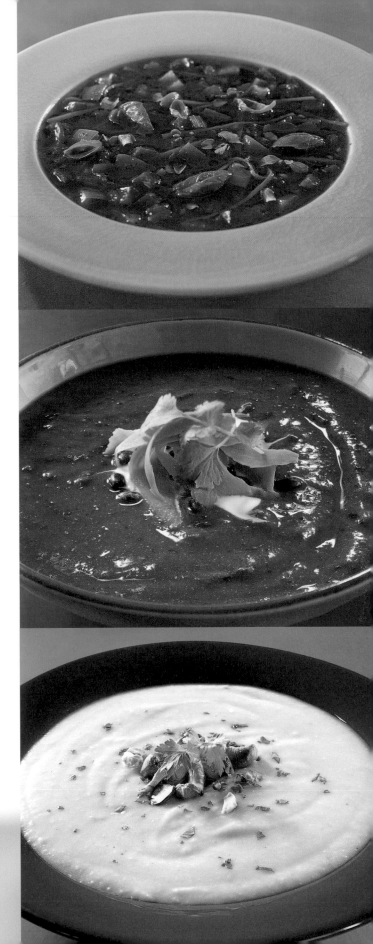

Basic Vegetable Soup

The variations on this basic theme are endless. In winter, root vegetables, such as parsnips, turnips, and rutabagas, make a grounding, warming soup base. In the summer, lighter greens can be substituted, along with fresh herbs. This is an easy soup to make for any number of people. For a stronger flavor, add one bay leaf per four people with the vegetables. The ingredients below are for one person; simply multiply them by the number of people you want to feed. Recipe per person

2 ounces mixed vegetables (celery, zucchini, carrots, turnips, rutabagas, potatoes)
½ tablespoon oil or butter (optional)
1 cup water

Sea salt or tamari to taste
Chopped parsley or cilantro, to garnish (optional)

1 Clean the vegetables and dice or slice attractively.

2 If liked, heat the oil or butter in a pan and sauté the mixed vegetables until they are slightly softer.

3 Place the water in a large pan or stockpot and bring to a boil. Add the vegetables, lower the heat, cover, and simmer for 20 minutes.

4 Season with tamari or sea salt, and serve garnished with chopped parsley or cilantro.

• **Blended Vegetable Soup:** After cooking, transfer the soup to a food processor or blender and purée it until smooth. Return it to the pan and heat through. Serve garnished with parsley or cilantro.

• **Hearty Vegetable Soup:** Legumes can be soaked, added to the wate,r and cooked until almost soft before adding the vegetables.

• **Spring Vegetable Soup:** For each person, add 1 ounce seasonal greens, such as sorrel, spinach, dandelion, or watercress, or 3 tablespoons chopped fresh herbs, such as basil, fennel, dill, or tarragon, to the soup before seasoning it. Cook for 5 minutes longer and then season with sea salt or tamari.

• **Creamy Vegetable Soup:** Replace some of the water with milk or soy milk; do this toward the end of the cooking because milk or soy milk should not be boiled but only heated. Alternatively, add 1 to 2 tablespoons cream or yogurt per person before serving.

• **Creamy Vegan Soup:** For each person, sauté 1 tablespoon rolled oats with the chopped vegetables. This makes a light, creamy, nourishing soup.

Winter Warming Soup

This variation of Basic Vegetable Soup (see left) is transformed into a hearty meal by adding barley, a wonderful aid to the digestive system and, when combined with warming spices, makes the perfect soup to counteract the winter cold. Use high-fiber whole grain hulled barley rather than pearl barley. Serves 6 to 8

3 tablespoons oil
4 sticks of celery, finely chopped
4 carrots, chopped into bite-size cubes
1 small rutabaga, chopped into bite-size cubes
2 quarts boiling water
2 bay leaves
½ cup hulled barley

1 teaspoon ground cumin
1 teaspoon ground coriander
½ teaspoon pepper
Sea salt to taste
1 tablespoon chopped fresh parsley
    or cilantro

1 Heat the oil in a large pan. Add the celery and sauté for 2 minutes. Add the carrots and rutabaga and continue cooking for 5 minutes longer.

2 Add the water, bay leaves, barley, and ground cumin and coriander. Simmer for 30 minutes, or until the vegetables and barley are soft.

3 Remove half the soup and purée it in a food processor or blender until smooth. Return it to the pan, and season with the pepper and salt. Reheat, then serve at once, garnished with the chopped parsley or cilantro.

Carrot Soup

Traditionally, orange or saffron-color symbolizes the fire of renunciation by which all karma (past action) is burned. In this vibrant soup, the orange juice and fresh mint lighten the earthy quality of the carrots. Serves 4 to 6

2 tablespoons butter or margarine
5½ cups grated carrots
2¼ cups water

2¼ cups orange juice
Salt and pepper
2 tablespoons chopped fresh mint

1 Melt the butter or margarine in a large pan and sauté the carrots until they begin to soften. Add the water, half cover, and simmer over low to medium heat for about 20 minutes, until the carrots are soft.

2 Remove from the heat and leave to cool slightly. Place the carrots and cooking water in a food processor or blender, add the orange juice, and purée the mixture until smooth. Alternatively, press through a large strainer.

3 Return the soup to the pan, season to taste with salt and pepper, and reheat without boiling. Serve garnished with the chopped mint.

• Omit the orange juice and double the quantity of water. Replace the chopped mint with a pinch of freshly grated nutmeg.

Nutty Parsnip Soup

As warm and comforting as it is unusual, this recipe was devised by Stephen Cooke, one of our guest chefs, who has since returned to Australia. The peanut butter adds body to the soothing, almost applelike sweetness of the parsnips. Serves 4 to 6

2 carrots, chopped	1½ quarts water
2 sticks of celery, chopped	1 to 2 tablespoons crunchy peanut butter
3 parsnips, chopped	Salt or tamari
1 tablespoon fresh thyme or cilantro leaves	Squeeze of lemon juice (optional)

1 Place the vegetables in a large pan with the herbs and water. Bring to a boil, half cover, and simmer for 15 to 20 minutes, until the vegetables are soft.

2 Leave to cool slightly, then transfer to a food processor or blender. Add the peanut butter and blend until smooth.

3 Return the purée to the pan. Season to taste with salt or tamari and add a little lemon juice, if desired. Reheat without boiling and serve at once.

Roasted Tomato Soup

Simple wholesome, pure foods like this soup help to maintain physical health and mental equilibrium. Try to use ripe red tomatoes, although the grated carrot guarantees whatever tomatoes you use the soup will not be too tart. Roasting the tomatoes first adds an exotic flavor to the soup. Serves 4 to 6

1 pound tomatoes	1 tablespoon torn fresh basil or 1 teaspoon dried
2 tablespoons oil	3⅓ cups hot water
1 red bell pepper, cored, seeded, and chopped	1 teaspoon salt
1 carrot, grated	¼ teaspoon pepper
2 sticks of celery, sliced	Basil and oregano leaves, or 2 tablespoons
1 tablespoon chopped fresh oregano or	chopped fresh parsley, to garnish
¾ teaspoon dried	

1 Heat the oven to 400°F and roast the whole tomatoes, turning them frequently until the skins fall away, about 15 minutes. Cool slightly, then peel and chop them.

2 Heat the oil in a pan and sauté the bell pepper, carrot, and celery over medium heat for a few minutes. Add the oregano and basil, stir well, and cook for a few minutes longer.

3 Add the water and tomatoes. Season with salt and pepper. Half cover and simmer for about 20 minutes. Transfer to a food processor or blender and blend for a few seconds. Return the soup to the pan and reheat if necessary, then serve garnished with fresh basil and oregano leaves or chopped parsley.

- For a thicker consistency, add 1½ cups chopped cooked potatoes to the vegetables.
- For an even heartier soup, add some cooked grain 10 minutes before the end of the cooking time.
- For a creamier soup, add a little soy milk or cream just before serving.

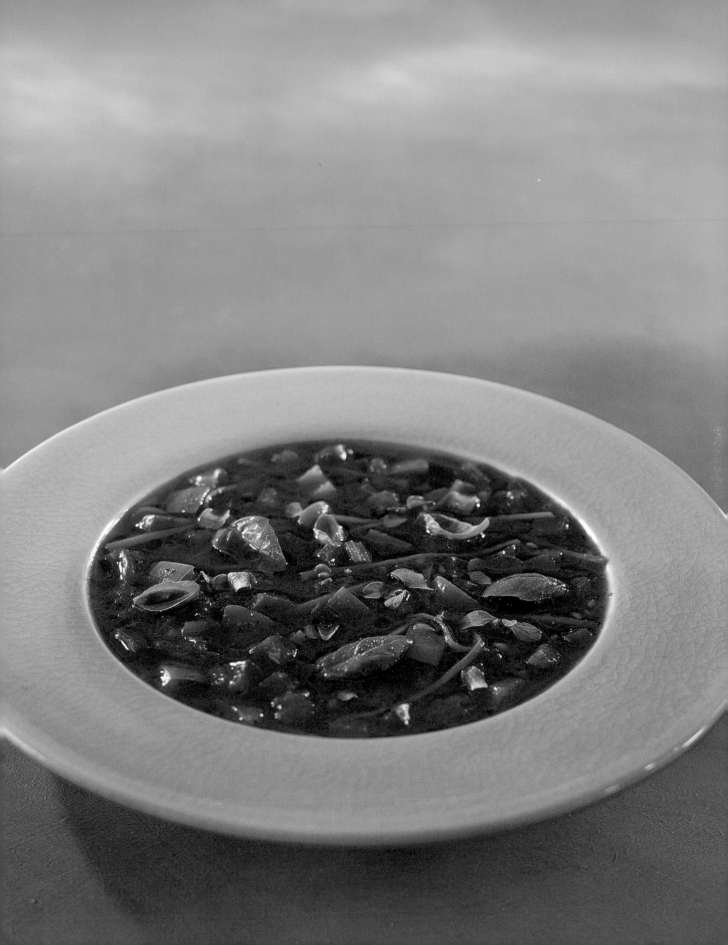

Borscht

A native dish from Eastern Europe, borscht can be served as either a summer or winter soup. When the temperature drops, serve the soup with a plate of boiled potatoes for a satisfying supper. Beets are an excellent blood tonic. Serves 6 to 8

1 tablespoon oil
1 stick of celery, chopped
1 bay leaf
4 raw beets, scrubbed and chopped into bite-size pieces
1 carrot, grated
1 potato, chopped into bite-size pieces
2¼ quarts water
1¾ cups chopped beet tops, spinach, or kale (optional)

Juice of ½ lemon
1 teaspoon salt
Pinch of pepper
Pinch of paprika
1 teaspoon fresh dill or ¼ teaspoon dried dillweed
Sour cream, soy cream, or plain yogurt, to serve
Finely chopped fresh parsley, to garnish

1 Heat the oil in a large pan and sauté the chopped celery until soft. Add the bay leaf, beets, carrot, potato, and water. Cover and simmer for about 45 minutes, until the beets are tender. Add the greens and cook for 10 minutes longer. Add the lemon juice, salt, pepper, paprika, and dill.

2 Serve hot, topped with a spoonful of sour cream, soy cream, or yogurt and garnished with chopped parsley.

• **Beet Soup with Tomatoes:** Add 1½ cups chopped tomatoes and 1 cinnamon stick with the greens. Omit the paprika and dill. Garnish with mint instead of parsley.

• **Cold Summer Borscht:** Prepare the soup ahead of time. Remove the bay leaf. Season, adding double the amount of lemon juice. Blend to a purée and chill. Spoon into individual bowls and serve with a spoonful of yogurt, sour cream, or soy cream on the top.

Golden Cauliflower Soup

If you have ever had the good fortune to stay at the Sivananda Ashram in Kerala, South India, the wonderful combination of cumin, turmeric, and coconut will evoke memories of that happy time. This is a superb recipe if you are planning an Indian-style meal. Be careful to not overcook the cumin—the delicate flavor can be easily lost if toasted for too long. Serves 4 to 6

1 cauliflower
1 tablespoon butter or margarine
1 tablespoon cumin seeds
½ teaspoon turmeric
2 or 3 potatoes, peeled and roughly chopped

4½ cups water
1 tablespoon unsweetened dried coconut, soaked in enough hot water to cover
Salt and pepper

1 Break the cauliflower into small flowerets and chop the stalk; set aside. Melt the butter or margarine in a large pan. Add the cumin seeds and toast for 1 minute, or until you smell the aroma. Lower the heat, add the cauliflower and turmeric, and sauté for 5 minutes, stirring well to make sure the flowerets are coated with turmeric. Remove half of the flowerets with a slotted spoon and set aside.

2 Add the potatoes and water to the pan and simmer for 15 minutes. Cool slightly, then purée the soup in a food processor or blender until smooth. Return it to the pan and stir in the coconut and its soaking water. Add the reserved cauliflower flowerets and simmer for 5 minutes longer. Season to taste with salt and pepper and serve at once.

Celery Root and Cashew Soup *This makes a perfect winter soup for festive meals such as Thanksgiving and Christmas.* Serves 6 to 8

1 tablespoon butter or margarine
3 cups chopped celery root
4 sticks of celery
⅔ cup cashew nuts
4½ cups water

1 potato, chopped
2¼ cups soy milk
Salt and pepper to taste
Toasted cashew nuts and parsley sprigs,
    to garnish

1 Melt the butter or margarine in a heavy pan and sauté the celery root, celery, and nuts over medium heat until they are lightly brown.

2 Add the water and potato, cover, and cook over medium heat for 25 minutes, until all the vegetables are tender.

3 Add the soy milk and purée in a food processor or blender. Season with salt and pepper. Return the soup to the pan and heat slowly until warm. Serve at once, garnished with toasted cashew nuts and parsley sprigs.

Vichyssoise *Among foods, potatoes are well known for their grounding energy; among asanas, it is the balancing exercises (crow, peacock, tree) that have that distinction. Traditionally served cold as a delightful summer soup, this version can also be heated (be careful not to boil the milk or soy milk) without any loss of flavor.* Serves 6

3 cups peeled and diced potatoes
1½ cups diced turnips
1 stick of celery, chopped
2 tablespoons butter or oil
2¼ cups water

1¾ cups milk or soy milk, plus extra if
    necessary
3 to 4 tablespoons finely chopped fresh parsley
½ teaspoon salt
Pepper to taste

1 Put the potatoes, turnips, and celery in a large pan with the butter or oil and the water, adding a little more water if necessary to cover the vegetables. Cover the pan and simmer the vegetables for 15 to 20 minutes, until they are soft.

2 Transfer the vegetables and the cooking water to a food processor or blender, add the 1¾ cups milk or soy milk, and purée until smooth.

3 Pour the soup into a large bowl and add more soy milk if necessary to bring the soup to the consistency you desire. Stir in the parsley and season with the salt and pepper. Chill for at least 1 hour before serving.

• **Vichyssoise with Cheese:** Substitute ½ cup grated vegetarian cheese or 1 ounce nutritional yeast flakes for some of the milk or soy milk. Serve hot, garnished with a little paprika.

• **Potage Cressonière:** After puréeing the soup, return it to the pan and add a generous 1 cup finely chopped watercress. Add ¼ teaspoon freshly grated nutmeg, if desired. Simmer for about 5 minutes, then stir in the soy milk. Alternatively, use 3 cups chopped spinach or young spring greens instead of the watercress. If using spring greens, season with paprika instead of nutmeg.

Corn Chowder
This hearty soup is quick and easy to make. Serve with a salad for a winter lunch, or as part of a festive meal. Serves 4 to 6

4 fresh ears of corn, or 3 cups canned corn kernels, drained	3 potatoes, chopped
1 tablespoon butter or margarine	2¼ cups soy milk
2 cups chopped celery, or 3½ cups cabbage	1 teaspoon salt
	Pepper

1 If using fresh corn, scrape off the kernels with a sharp knife.

2 Melt the butter or margarine in a large pan and sauté the celery or cabbage over medium heat for 5 minutes. Add the potatoes and fresh or canned corn kernels and cover with water. (You can add the cobs to the liquid while cooking to improve the flavor of the stock.) Half cover the pan and simmer until the corn is tender.

3 Transfer the soup to a food processor or blender, discarding the cobs if they have been added for flavoring, and blend to a coarse purée (the sweetcorn kernel skins will not blend to a smooth purée). Return the soup to the pan and add the soy milk and salt and pepper to taste. Reheat and serve at once.

• **Mexican Corn Chowder:** This chunky variation is a meal in itself. Replace the celery or cabbage with 1 red and 1 green bell pepper, cored, seeded, and chopped. Add 1 teaspoon ground cumin, 2 teaspoons dried oregano, and ¼ teaspoon cayenne pepper to the vegetables. Do not blend the soup and omit the soy milk. Serve hot, garnished with cilantro leaves. If liked, top each serving with diced vegetarian cheese.

Cuban Black Bean Soup
Not to be confused with black-eyed peas, black beans are small, matt-black beans, warming by nature and believed to help strengthen kidney energy. In this traditional Cuban recipe, their strong earthy flavor is perfectly complemented by the sweetness of the potatoes and the heat of the ginger. For a more substantial dish, serve with cooked brown rice, either stirred into the soup or served separately. To add extra color, garnish with strips of blanched sweet potato and parsley sprigs. Serves 4 to 6

1¾ cups dried black beans, soaked for 3 to 4 hours	1 tablespoon chopped fresh gingerroot (optional)
4½ cups water	2 tablespoons butter or margarine
1 sweet potato or yam, diced	Salt
1 bay leaf	Yogurt, sour cream, or grated vegetarian cheese, to serve (optional)

1 Drain the beans and place them in a large pan with the water. Bring to a boil and boil vigorously for 10 minutes. Lower the heat.

2 Add the sweet potato or yam, bay leaf, and ginger, if using. Cover and simmer for about 1 hour, or until the beans are tender, adding more water if necessary. Leave to cool slightly, then purée in a food processor or blender until the soup is smooth (leave a few beans whole to stir into the purée, if preferred).

3 Return the purée to the pan and add the butter or margarine. Season to taste with salt. Simmer for 10 minutes. Serve at once, topped with yogurt, sour cream, or grated cheese, if desired.

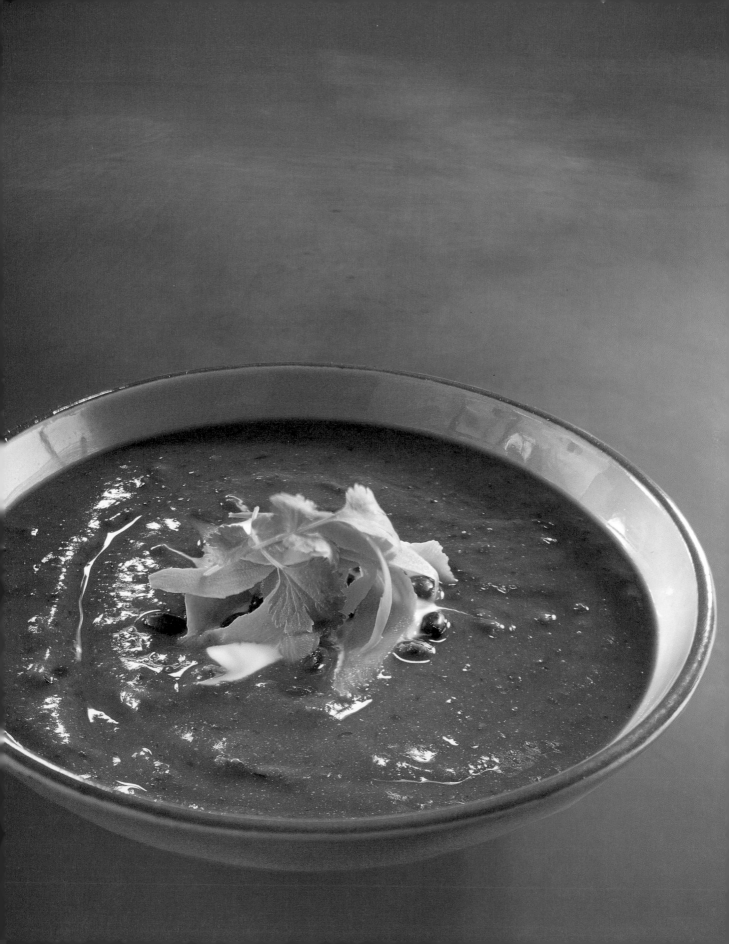

Lentil Soup
Rich in protein and iron, lentils are used in everything from light summery soups to hearty winter dishes. They do not need to be soaked, but soaking them for 30 minutes helps to remove the phytates that might impede the absorption of iron. Serves 6

1 to 2 tablespoons oil, butter, or ghee	2 bay leaves
2 carrots, diced	1 tablespoon tomato paste (optional)
1 medium rutabaga or turnip, diced	About 1½ quarts hot water
2 sticks of celery, chopped	1 teaspoon salt or 1 tablespoon tamari
2 cups lentils, soaked for 30 minutes	1 teaspoon each dried oregano and thyme

1 Heat the oil, butter, or ghee in a heavy-bottomed pan and sauté the carrots, rutabaga or turnip, and celery for 3 to 4 minutes. Drain the lentils and add them to the pan with the bay leaves, tomato paste, if using, and 4½ cups of the water. Bring to a boil, then reduce the heat, half cover, and simmer for 15 to 20 minutes, or until the lentils are soft.

2 Add the salt or tamari, oregano, thyme, and as much of the remaining water as is necessary to achieve the consistency of your choice. Simmer for 2 to 3 minutes and serve.

Split Pea Soup
This recipe is a winter favorite at the Sivananda Headquarters in Quebec, where temperatures often drop to -40°F. Serves 8

Generous 1 cup split peas (yellow or green)	1 teaspoon dried basil
1½ quarts water	½ teaspoon ground ginger
2 tablespoons oil, butter, or margarine	1 teaspoon ground cumin
2 carrots, sliced into thin rounds	1 teaspoon honey (optional)
2 sticks of celery, finely chopped	1 tablespoon lemon juice (optional)
2 potatoes, cut into large cubes	1 teaspoon salt and ¼ teaspoon pepper

1 Rinse the split peas and place them in a large pan with the water. Cover and simmer for about 40 minutes, until tender.

2 Heat the oil, butter, or margarine in a separate pan and sauté the vegetables with the herbs and spices over medium heat for 5 minutes. Add them to the cooked split peas. Bring back to a boil and simmer, covered, for 20 minutes longer, until the peas are very soft. Add the honey and lemon juice, if using. Season with the salt and pepper and serve at once.

Tofu-Vegetable Soup Orientale
A simple, delicate soup, this is ideal if you want a light, but flavorful course before heavier dishes. Serves 4 to 6

1 tablespoon oil	9 ounces firm tofu, cut into bite-size pieces
2 ounces water chestnuts, sliced	1½ quarts boiling water
2 ounces bamboo shoots, sliced	3 ounces trimmed and sliced snow peas
⅔ cup chopped kohlrabi	¼ cup tamari

1 Heat the oil in a large pan. Add the water chestnuts, bamboo shoots, kohlrabi, and tofu. Stir-fry for about 4 minutes.

2 Add the boiling water and simmer for 10 minutes. Add the snow peas and simmer for 2 to 3 minutes longer. Season with tamari and serve at once.

Miso A salty paste made from beans and/or grains, miso is mostly used to add flavor to soups and sauces. It is highly beneficial in the diet as a source of protein, and is reputed to have remarkable medicinal properties. In Japan it is used to cure colds, improve metabolism, clear the skin, and help develop resistance to parasitic diseases! Each type of miso adds a different flavor to food. It is best to buy organic miso at your local health-food store—you use so little, it is worth the expense. Light miso is fragrant and sweet. Red-brown miso is aromatic and tasty, and dark miso is pungent and salty. Never boil miso because it destroys the helpful microorganisms. Also, do not reheat miso soup because the heat destroys the nutritional value.

Miso Soup

Miso soup is warm and soothing on a cold day; refreshing on a hot day. This basic soup can be varied by adding grains or noodles. Serves 6

A few pieces of arame or wakame seaweed,
soaked in enough water to cover for 5 minutes
2 teaspoons sesame oil
6 ounces finely chopped or sliced vegetables
(cabbage, celery, carrots, rutabaga, turnip)

2 teaspoons grated fresh gingerroot
4½ cups water
4 tablespoons dark miso
2 tablespoons fresh parsley or cilantro leaves

1 Drain the arame or wakame and cut it into 1-inch strips; set aside. Heat the oil in a wok or heavy pan. Add the vegetables and ginger, and sauté for about 5 minutes.

2 Add the seaweed and water and bring to a boil. Half cover and simmer for 15 minutes. Remove from the heat. Mix the miso with a little of the soup, then stir it into the pan. Serve at once, garnished with parsley or cilantro.

Salmoreio

Elizabeth, the mother of one of our staff, contributed this recipe; it joined our repertory during one of our month-long yoga teachers' training courses in Spain. Prana-laden ripe tomatoes bring out the true character of this traditional chilled Andalusian soup. The amount of tomato juice depends on how thick you like the soup. Serve with fresh bread, rice cakes, or crudités. Serves 4 to 6

1 pound tomatoes, chopped
2 tablespoons chopped fresh basil
1 cup fresh bread crumbs
3 tablespoons extra-virgin olive oil
2 tablespoons lemon juice
1 tablespoon tomato paste

1 teaspoon chopped fresh gingerroot
½ teaspoon cayenne pepper
1 teaspoon salt
Pepper to taste
½ to 1 cup tomato juice or water

Put all the ingredients in a food processor or blender, adding ½ cup tomato juice or water. Blend until thick and smooth. Add the remaining tomato juice or water if the soup is too thick. Chill before serving.

• **Gazpacho:** Omit the ginger and half the bread crumbs. Add half a peeled and chopped cucumber, ½ a cored, seeded, and chopped green bell pepper, 1 chopped stick of celery, and 2 tablespoons finely chopped parsley. Use tomato juice rather than water. Blend and chill. To serve, add some ice cubes and garnish with chopped cucumber and pepper and/or whole wheat croutons.

GLORIOUS GRAINS

"Like grain, the mortal decays
And like grain, he is born again."

Katha Upanishad, I. 6

"Many people consider life as a straight line, from A to B, from birth to death. But yoga masters speak of a triangle. The first point represents birth; the line going upward represents growth. The top point represents youth; then the downward line is decay or old age, and at the end of decay is the last point, representing death. The bottom line represents life hereafter which leads us again to the first point, birth—reincarnation. Again there is growth; again youth, decay, death, and life hereafter, and then again birth. So life goes on and on and on, forever and ever and ever."

Swami Vishnu-devananda

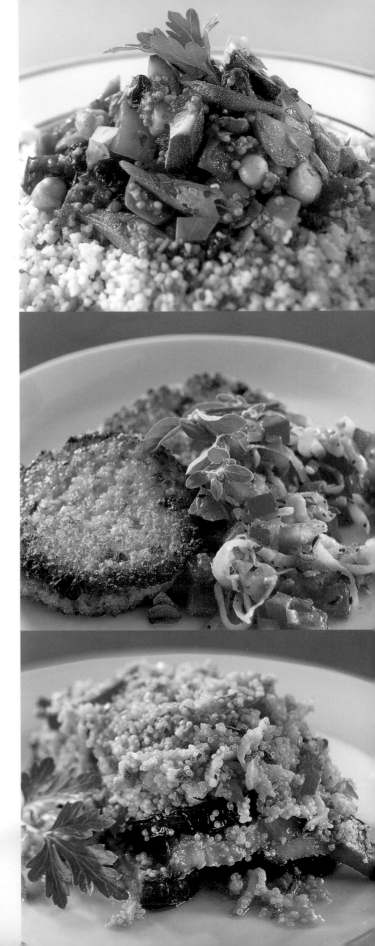

The yogic diet is essentially grain based. Whole grains are the primary source of carbohydrates, the origin of energy for the human body. Complex carbohydrates are abundant in nature, relatively inexpensive, and filling. Unrefined grains are rich in fiber and B vitamins and supply about half of the amino acids that form protein. They should be eaten every day, preferably with foods containing complementary proteins, such as legumes. Most of the world's population survives on a diet of legume and grain combinations.

Weigh or measure whole grains, then rinse them two or three times, until the water runs clear. Drain and put into a heavy saucepan, together with the appropriate amount of water (see chart below). Bring to a boil, reduce the heat, and simmer until all the water has been absorbed. The cooking times in the chart below include bringing the water to a boil.

Grains may be presoaked to reduce the cooking time. Alternatively, they may be dry roasted in the oven at 375°F for 15 to 30 minutes, or in a heated dry skillet over high heat for a few minutes, before boiling, to give them a sweet, nutty flavor.

COOKING GRAINS

The volume of water needed for cooking varies from twice to four-and-a-half times the volume of the grain.

Grain	Amount	Volume of water	Cooking time	Serves
Barley	1 cup	2½ times	1¼ hours	4 to 6
Buckwheat groats	1 cup	Twice	15 to 25 minutes	4 to 6
Bulgur	1 cup	Twice	Pour boiling water over and leave for 15 to 20 minutes	4 to 6
Cornmeal	1⅔ cups	3 to 3½ times	15 minutes	4 to 6
Couscous	1 cup	Twice	Pour boiling water over, cover, and leave 15 to 20 minutes	4 to 6
Millet	1 cup	2½ to 3 times	30 to 45 minutes	4 to 6
Oats, rolled	1¼ cups	2½ to 3 times	15 to 30 minutes	2 to 3
Quinoa	1 cup	Twice	15 minutes	4
Rice, basmati	1 cup	Twice	20 to 35 minutes	4 to 6
Rice, brown	1 cup	2 to 2½ times	40 to 50 minutes	4
Rye grains	1 cup	3½ times	2 hours	4
Wheat berries	1 cup	4½ times	45 to 60 minutes	4 to 6

Rice One of the great staples of the world, rice features heavily in the yogic diet. In Asia, rice is the emblem of prosperity (both material and spiritual), happiness, and nourishment. In India, rice is sacred and is used in all rituals. When guests arrive they are asked "Have you had your rice?" as the first duty to the guest is to offer him or her food. Rice has a balancing effect on the entire digestive system and soothes the nervous system. Because it is neither heating nor cooling to the system, rice can be combined with herbs and spices in a myriad of ways to harmonize imbalances in the body. Short-grain brown rice offers the richest source of vitamins and minerals. Most popular in Ayurveda, basmati rice is a light and aromatic long-grain variety with a cooling effect on the body. It is good for calming an irritated gut and is easier to digest than brown rice.

To cook brown rice, rinse the rice first, then cook in a heavy-bottomed saucepan with a tight-fitting lid. The general rule is one measure of rice to two or two-and-a-half measures of cold water. Bring to a boil, then reduce the heat, cover the pan, and simmer for 40 to 50 minutes; do not remove the lid during this time as the steam plays an essential part in the cooking process. After about 45 minutes the water will have been absorbed and the rice will be tender with a delicious, chewy texture. Another way to cook rice is to gently toast it in a dry pan for a few minutes, then add the water and cook as above.

To cook basmati rice, rinse it in cold water to remove much of the starch, changing the water until the water is clear. Bring just under twice the volume of water to rice to the boil, add the rice and a pinch of salt to taste, reduce the heat, cover, and cook for 10 to 15 minutes, by which time all the water should be absorbed. Remove the pan from the heat and leave to stand for 5 minutes before removing the lid.

Rice Pilau
Basmati is the rice considered to be the best among the many Indian varieties—its name means "queen of fragrance"—and is the one most often used in festive Indian dishes. Brown basmati rice contains more nutrients than the white variety. Rice pilau can be used along with dal to make a simple meal, or can be used as part of a more elaborate meal. Serves 4 to 6

1½ cups basmati rice
4 tablespoons ghee or vegetable oil
⅓ cup raw cashews, almonds, or pistachio nuts, chopped
1 teaspoon cumin seeds
¾-inch piece of fresh gingerroot, peeled and shredded

1 or 2 green chilies, seeded and finely chopped
2½ cups hot water
1 cup fresh peas or finely sliced green beans
½ teaspoon garam masala
1 teaspoon salt
⅓ cup raisins (optional)

1 Rinse the rice and soak in cold water for 15 to 20 minutes, then drain. Heat the ghee or oil in a heavy pan over low heat. Add the nuts and sauté, stirring constantly, until golden brown. Remove from the oil.

2 Increase the heat to medium. Add the cumin seeds, ginger, and chilies to the pan and cook until the cumin is golden brown, stirring constantly. Stir in the rice and stir-fry for 2 minutes. Add the hot water, peas, garam masala, salt, and raisins, if using. Bring to a boil, then reduce the heat to very low, cover with a tight-fitting lid, and simmer for 10 to 15 minutes, until all the water is absorbed and the rice is tender and fluffy. Serve at once.

Rice Salad

Poornima, the full moon night, is considered by yogis to be especially auspicious for spiritual practice. Guru Poornima, the full moon around mid-July, is dedicated to the teacher. It is the occasion of the London center's annual boat trip on the River Thames, complete with chanting and a feast. This recipe, which may be prepared in advance, is usually one of the highlights of the celebration. It is served along with other salads (pages 96 to 99) and items from the Middle Eastern Feast (page 142). Serves 8

1½ cups long-grain brown or basmati rice
2½ cups water
6 tablespoons olive oil
3 tablespoons lemon juice
2 tablespoons chopped fresh herbs, such as parsley, basil, mint, lemon balm

1 pound mixed vegetables, such as blanched asparagus or peas, avocado, bell pepper, carrot, celery, cucumber, fennel, and pitted olives, diced if necessary
1 teaspoon salt
¼ teaspoon pepper

1 Place the rice in a heavy pan with the water. Bring to a boil, cover, and simmer for 35 to 40 minutes for brown rice or 20 to 35 minutes for basmati rice, until all the water is absorbed.

2 Leave the rice to cool. Toss the cooked rice, olive oil, and lemon juice gently with a fork (a spoon tends to mash the rice). Stir in the herbs and diced vegetables. Season with the salt and pepper.

3 Rice salad can be served right away, but it tastes best if the flavors are left to blend for about 2 hours. Serve each portion on a lettuce leaf or in a hollowed-out tomato or bell pepper. Alternatively, press into a lightly greased mold and chill in the refrigerator for several hours before turning out.

• **Seeded Rice Salad:** Replace the vegetables and herbs with 2 teaspoons sesame seeds, 2 tablespoons sunflower seeds, and 2 tablespoons pumpkin seeds, each toasted separately. Substitute 3 tablespoons tahini for the olive oil.

Congee

Yogis have traditionally eaten this rice soup for thousands of years, as it is easy to prepare, nutritious, and tastes good. It is the favorite evening meal at our Sivananda Yoga Vedanta Nataraja Center in New Delhi, especially in wintertime. A popular breakfast or supper dish throughout Asia, congee (also known as kanji) is a very calming food that soothes and strengthens the digestion, and for this reason it is often given to invalids or children. Serves 4 to 6

1 cup brown rice
1-inch piece fresh gingerroot, peeled and sliced or chopped

3⅓ quarts water
Salt, tamari, or Gomasio (page 118) to taste, or nori, toasted and crumbled

1 Place the rice and ginger in a heavy pan with the water. Bring to a boil, cover, and cook over medium heat for about 1 hour, until the rice breaks down to a soupy consistency. Remove the pan from the heat and spoon the soup into individual bowls.

2 Season to taste with salt, tamari, or gomasio, or sprinkle toasted and crumbled nori over the top, and serve at once.

Stir-Fried Rice with Bean Sprouts *The ever-popular Chinese stir-fry is fast, easy, and a full meal in itself.* Serves 4 to 6

3 tablespoons oil
2 teaspoons grated or chopped fresh gingerroot
1 red bell pepper, cored, seeded, and coarsely chopped
1¾ cups bean sprouts (either mung or soy)
3½ cups shredded cabbage
7 ounces water chestnuts, sliced

7 ounces bamboo shoots, sliced
4 ounces baby corn
4 ounces snow peas, sliced into 1-inch pieces
9 ounces firm tofu, cubed or broken
Generous 2 cups cooked rice
Tamari

1 Heat the oil in a wok or heavy skillet and stir-fry the ginger for about 1 minute. Add the chopped bell pepper and stir-fry for 2 minutes.

2 Add the other vegetables and the tofu and stir-fry for 2 minutes longer. Stir in the cooked rice and mix well. Remove from the heat and add tamari to taste. Serve at once.

Paella *The traditional Spanish dish, is given a yogic "twist" by using brown rice and arame, one of the milder tasting sea vegetables. Like all sea vegetables, arame has a cooling effect and helps to cleanse the body of toxins. It is important to soak sea vegetables in water to remove the excess salt before using. This paella makes a delicious meal served with a green salad.* Serves 6

1½ cups brown rice
2½ cups water
10 ounces firm tofu, cut into cubes
4 tablespoons tamari
2 tablespoons arame seaweed, soaked in enough water to cover for about 5 minutes
Oil for deep-frying
1 eggplant, halved lengthwise and thinly sliced

2 tablespoons olive oil
2 carrots, sliced diagonally
1 red bell pepper, cored, seeded, and cut into strips
1 teaspoon turmeric
3 to 4 tablespoons lemon juice
24 pitted ripe olives
2 tablespoons chopped fresh parsley

1 Put the brown rice in a heavy pan and add the water. Bring to a boil, lower the heat, cover, and simmer for 35 to 40 minutes, until all the water is absorbed and the rice is tender.

2 Meanwhile, marinate the tofu in the tamari for 30 minutes; drain. Drain the arame.

3 Heat the oil for frying in a heavy skillet. Add the eggplant slices and tofu cubes, a few at a time, and cook until sealed and crispy. Drain on paper towels.

4 Heat the olive oil in the skillet. Add the carrots, red bell pepper, and turmeric and sauté until the vegetables are tender. Stir in the cooked rice and lemon juice. Gently fold in the tofu cubes, eggplant, and arame. Garnish with the ripe olives and chopped parsley and serve hot.

Baked Rice

Sankar and Tejas, our "men in Toronto," sent in this recipe along with the following comments: "This is a grain recipe we have made quite a few times. We really like it because it is simple, tasty, and the rice is very well cooked, so it's much easier to digest. It's great with stir-fry veggies. Good cooking!!!" Serves 4 to 6

3 teaspoons hijiki seaweed, soaked in enough water to cover for 15 minutes
⅔ cup chopped raw cashew nuts
1 tablespoon oil
2 carrots, cut into matchsticks
3½ cups finely shredded cabbage

½ cup cubed eggplant
1¼ cups brown rice
½ cup red lentils
3⅓ cups water
⅔ cup sliced fresh peas or green beans
1 teaspoon salt

1 Drain the hijiki. Toast the cashew nuts in a hot, dry skillet until brown; remove from the pan and set aside. Heat the oil in a large pan and sauté the carrots, cabbage, and eggplant over medium heat for 5 to 7 minutes, until softened slightly. Stir in the rice and sauté for 1 minute. Add the hijiki and sauté lightly for a few moments. Add the lentils and water. Bring to a boil, lower the heat, cover tightly, and cook over low heat for about 30 minutes.

2 Meanwhile, heat the oven to 350°F. Uncover the pan and, if necessary, add another ¼ to ½ cup water along with the peas or beans, salt, and cashews. Transfer to a greased baking dish, cover, and bake in the oven for about 20 minutes. Serve hot.

Quinoa Quinoa (pronounced keen-wa) is an ancient grain making a come-back. It has a high amino acid content, is easy to cook and digest, and is gluten-free, making it a great alternative for people with corn or wheat allergies. It can be substituted for rice or millet in most recipes. Quinoa must be washed thoroughly; place in a fine mesh strainer and rinse until the water runs clear.

Eggplant-Quinoa Roast

This high-energy grain from South America's Andes mountains is given an international flavor in this vegetable-rich dish, needing only a green salad to complement it. Serves 4

4 tablespoons sesame oil
12 ounces eggplant, cut into 8 thick slices
2 tablespoons tamari
¼ cup lemon juice
½ cup water

1 teaspoon grated fresh gingerroot
1 cup quinoa, washed
1 large red bell pepper, cored, seeded, and sliced
2 zucchini, coarsely grated
Parsley sprigs, to garnish

1 Heat the oven to 350°F. Heat the sesame oil in a skillet and cook the eggplant slices until brown. Arrange them in a single layer in a baking dish. Combine the tamari, lemon juice, water, and ginger and pour over the eggplant slices. Bake in the oven for 10 minutes. Turn the slices over and cook for 10 minutes longer, until most of the liquid is absorbed.

2 Place the quinoa in a large pan with double its volume of water. Bring to a boil, cover, and simmer for 15 minutes, until tender. Drain if necessary. Add the red bell pepper and zucchini to the sesame oil remaining in the skillet and sauté until soft. Add the quinoa, mix well, and spoon over the eggplant. Press down well. Return to the oven and bake for 5 to 10 minutes longer. Serve hot, garnished with parsley sprigs.

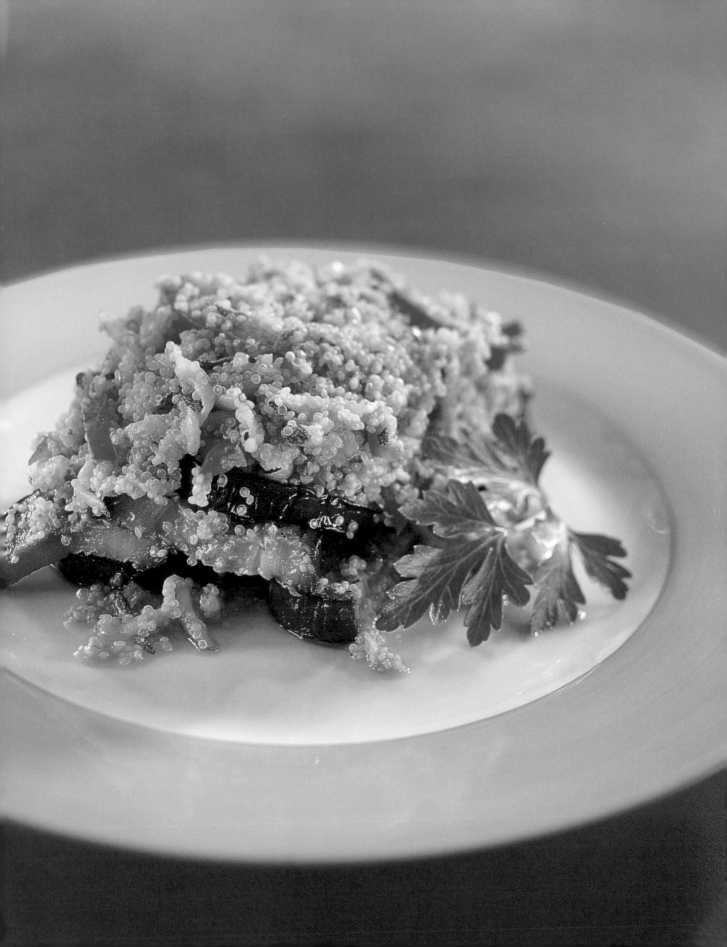

Wheat Rich in vitamins and minerals, whole wheat is an essential ingredient in a yogi's diet, eaten as a grain, made into pasta, or used as flour for bread. It is important to avoid refined wheat as most of the energy-giving nutrients of the grain have been removed. Wheat has a cooling effect on the system and can help to reduce inflammation. It also stimulates the liver to cleanse itself. Wheat allergies are very common, but usually they are an allergic reaction to the quantity and quality of the processed wheat most of us eat; organically grown whole wheat is less likely to cause a reaction. Gluten is a protein in wheat flour which traps air in dough and makes bread rise. It is also found in rye and barley, but in smaller quantities. If you find wheat, or these other grains, cause bloating, gas, stomach pain, indigestion, or excessive mucus, do not eat them, especially during pregnancy. Rice, millet, quinoa, or spelt may be substituted. Most people with wheat sensitivities find they can easily tolerate rye and barley—and organically grown wheat does not disturb them.

Spelt is an ancient relative of wheat enjoying a renewed popularity. Spelt can usually be tolerated by people with wheat and gluten sensitivities. Higher in protein and fiber than most varieties of wheat, spelt is available in health-food stores in the form of pastas, flour, breads, and whole grains. It may be substituted for wheat in any recipe, using the same quantities.

Whole Wheat Bread

Our daily bread, more than any other food, symbolizes the giving of human, as well as divine, love. Eating bread can be a mystical as well as communal experience. Fresh bread baked with love has the mysterious power of bringing warmth and togetherness into any home or gathering. God is everywhere, but the daily ritual of the breaking of bread can serve to bring that awareness to mind. Chew the bread well and think of the many blessings you have. Many people in the world have neither enough food to eat nor clean water to drink. They do not have a healthy body to enable them to work out their karma. In the words of Swami Sivananda: "The first wealth is health. It is the greatest of all possessions. It is the basis of all virtues. The person with health has hope, and he who has hope has everything." Makes 2 loaves, about 2 pounds each

2 tablespoons active-dry yeast	3 tablespoons barley malt syrup
1 quart lukewarm water	3 pounds 5 ounces (12½ cups) whole wheat flour
¼ cup oil	2 teaspoons sea salt

1 Sprinkle the yeast into the water in a bowl and leave in a warm place for 10 minutes. Add the oil, barley malt syrup, and half the flour and blend well. Cover and leave to rise for 30 minutes.

2 Stir in the rest of the flour and the salt and knead to a smooth dough, adding a little more flour if necessary (the dough should not be too sticky). Leave to rise again for 45 to 60 minutes, until doubled in size.

3 Punch down the risen dough to knock out any large air bubbles, shape into two loaves, and place in two lightly greased 9- x 5-inch bread pans. Leave to rise until the top of the center of the dough is level with the top of the pans; do not let it over rise or the dough will crack. Meanwhile, heat the oven to 450°F. Bake in the oven on the top shelf for 15 minutes. Reduce the heat to 375°F and bake for 1 hour longer. Leave to cool before serving—hot bread tastes great but it is difficult to digest.

- **Poppy Seed Bread:** Add to the basic mix 4 tablespoons poppy seeds, 1 teaspoon almond extract, and 1 tablespoon raisins or finely chopped dates.
- **Seed Bread:** Add 2 tablespoons each of poppy seeds, sesame seeds, sunflower seeds, and pumpkin seeds with the flour.
- **Sesame-Honey Bread:** Use sesame oil in the basic mix and add $2/3$ cup sesame seeds and 1 to 2 tablespoons honey.
- **Oat Bread:** Reduce the amount of whole wheat flour to 2 pounds 14 ounces ($10^3/4$ cups). Add $2^1/2$ cups rolled oats, or $2/3$ cup cornmeal and 1 cup plus 2 tablespoons rolled oats.
- **Rye Bread:** Reduce the amount of whole wheat flour to $6^1/4$ cups and add $7^1/2$ cups unsifted rye flour and 1 tablespoon crushed caraway seeds.

Chapatis

This is the basic flat bread served throughout northern India, always cooked fresh for each meal. One of the great delights of Sivananda Kutir, our small Himalayan ashram, is to sit on the kitchen veranda and be served hot, freshly made chapatis. Just in front, the Ganges River roars by; overhead, the eagles soar. Chapatis are the staple food of northern India, as rice is in the south. They are the "spoon" of the meal. To eat, break off a piece of chapati (with the right hand) and use it to scoop up vegetables, dal, pickle and yogurt, or raita. Makes about 18

2 cups plus ½ tablespoon whole wheat flour
1 teaspoon salt

About ¾ cup water
Ghee or oil for brushing (optional)

1 Combine the flour and salt in a bowl. Gradually stir in the water until the dough binds together, but is not sticky or wet. Knead well for about 10 minutes, until firm and elastic. Grease a bowl, turn the dough in it twice, then cover with a damp dish towel. Leave to sit for 1 hour, then knead again.

2 Form the dough into $1/2$ inch diameter balls. Flatten them and roll into discs about $1/8$ inch thick, using a greased rolling pin. As you do this, roll the chapati a couple of times and turn it slightly; repeat the turning as you roll to prevent the chapati sticking to the board. Make sure each chapati is symmetrical so it puffs up well.

3 Cook in a very hot, ungreased pan over high heat for a few seconds on each side, until lightly brown. Using a damp cloth, press on each side to make the bread puff up in the center. Brush the chapatis lightly with ghee or oil, if desired, and pile them up as you make them, wrapping them in a damp cloth until ready to serve.

- **Puris:** Deep-fry the chapatis in hot oil, pressing down once with the back of a large, metal spoon to puff them up. These are better than chapatis for a feast, because they can be cooked in advance.
- **Paratha:** Follow the chapati recipe. Roll out the dough, making sure it is symmetrical. Brush the top with melted ghee; dust with flour. Pleat the edges until a fist-size package forms; flatten and roll out again. Turn it over and do the same on the other side. The more times you do this, the flakier the paratha will be—twice is the minimum. Cook on a very hot, ungreased pan for a few seconds, brush with a little ghee, and flip it over. Repeat on the other side. It is ready when lightly brown. Parathas may be stuffed with any curried vegetable: served with yogurt they are a typical breakfast or evening meal in northern India.

Banana Bread

Half cake, half bread, but doubly good—even better spread with butter—is the unanimous verdict of the London Sivanada Yoga Centre. Banana breads tend to be moist, so they must be baked in well regulated ovens, otherwise the outside will be overbaked before the inside is ready. If you have this problem, get your oven checked, or try baking at a lower temperature. Makes 1 loaf

3 very ripe bananas
⅓ cup honey
1⅔ cups whole wheat flour
½ teaspoon salt

1 teaspoon baking soda
2 tablespoons butter, melted, or oil
¾ cup chopped nuts (optional)

1 Heat the oven to 350°F. Purée the bananas in a food processor or blender, or mash them with a fork. Add the honey and blend again or mix with a whisk. Sift the flour, salt, and baking soda together. Add the flour to the honey and banana mixture and stir with a whisk to combine everything. Add the butter or oil and the nuts, if using.

2 Pour into a 9 x 5-inch greased bread pan and bake for about 1 hour. To check it is baked, press lightly with a finger to see if the bread pops up, or insert a toothpick into the center to see if it comes out clean. Cool on a wire rack.

Peaceful Pizza

This recipe comes from Ganesha, our Yogi of the North. He is probably the best vegetarian pizza maker, and definitely the best yoga teacher, in Scotland. If you have a wheat allergy, substitute spelt flour for the wheat flour. The variety of toppings is infinite. Serves 4 to 8

Crust:
2½ cups hard white flour
½ envelop (⅛ ounce) quick-rise yeast
1 tablespoon olive oil
2 teaspoons turbinado sugar
½ teaspoon sea salt
About ¾ cup water (120°F)

Topping:
1 quantity of Tomato Sauce (page 123)
1 cup grated vegetarian cheese, or tahini
2 red or yellow bell peppers (or 1 of each), cored, seeded, and sliced (optional)
12 olives (optional)
Olive oil for drizzling

1 To make the crust, combine all the ingredients, except the water, in a bowl. Gradually add the water, mixing by hand until the dough forms a slightly sticky ball; the exact amount of water will depend on the flour used.

2 Turn out the dough onto a floured board and knead well for about 10 minutes, adding a little more flour if necessary. Alternatively, mix in a food processor until a slightly sticky dough forms, then turn out and knead for about 1 minute. Put the dough into a lightly greased mixing bowl, cover with a cloth, and leave to rise in a warm place for about 1 hour, or until double in size.

3 Heat the oven to 450°F. Divide the dough in half. Knead each portion into a ball, then roll out to fit two lightly greased 13- x 10-inch baking sheets. Place the dough on the baking sheets. Divide the tomato sauce between the pizzas and spread out evenly. Sprinkle the cheese over the sauce. Decorate with peppers and olives, if using, and a drizzle of olive oil. Bake the pizzas in the oven for about 15 minutes, then swop them over if they are on separate shelves in the oven and bake for 5 to 10 minutes longer, until the crusts are lightly brown.

Whole Wheat Spaghetti with Miso Sauce

An unusual and delicious recipe blending East-West cuisines, but remember noodles originated in Asia. For the miso sauce, use red ake miso or dark hatcho miso (see Glossary, page 156). If possible, make the sauce 6 to 8 hours in advance to let the flavors blend. Serves 4 to 6

2 tablespoons oil
2 sticks of celery, finely chopped
⅔ cup chopped fennel
3 tomatoes, diced
3 green bell peppers, cored, seeded, and diced
½ carrot, grated
1¾ cups water
4 bay leaves

5 tablespoons miso
1 tablespoon butter or margarine
1 tablespoon chopped fresh basil
Pepper to taste
18 ounces whole wheat spaghetti
Grated cheese or nutritional yeast
   flakes for sprinkling (optional)

1 Heat the oil in a heavy pan and sauté the celery and fennel over medium heat for about 10 minutes. Add the tomatoes, green bell peppers, and carrot and sauté for 15 minutes longer.

2 Add the water and bay leaves. Bring to a boil, lower the heat, and simmer, uncovered, for 10 minutes. Remove from the heat and stir in the miso, butter or margarine, and basil. Season to taste with pepper.

3 Cook the spaghetti in boiling water until *al dente* (tender but still firm to the bite). Drain well. Remove the bay leaves from the sauce and stir in the hot spaghetti. Add the cheese or yeast flakes, if using, and serve at once.

• Add 5 to 7 ounces cubed tofu when you add the vegetables.

Vegetarian Lasagne
There are many ways to make lasagne. This one is a favorite of Swami Mahadevananda, the Italian-born director of the Sivananda Dhanwanthari Ashram in Kerala, South India. Serve it with a green salad. Serves 4 to 6

6 ounces spinach, steamed and squeezed dry
9 ounces firm tofu, crumbled and drained
Salt and pepper
2 tablespoons olive oil
1 red bell pepper, cored, seeded, and cut into
   matchsticks

2 zucchini, cut into matchsticks
1 quantity of Tomato Sauce (page 123)
6 sheets of dried lasagne, cooked and drained
1 cup grated vegetarian cheese
2 tablespoons sunflower or sesame seeds
2 tablespoons nutritional yeast flakes (optional)

1 Heat the oven to 350°F. Chop the spinach and mix it with the tofu. Season with salt and pepper. Heat the oil and sauté the bell pepper and zucchini strips over medium heat for 3 minutes.

2 Spoon a layer of tomato sauce into an greased 10- x 8-inch baking dish. Cover this with a layer of cooked lasagne, then half the tofu and spinach mixture, and half the zucchini and bell pepper strips. Sprinkle with half the grated cheese.

3 Repeat the layers, then sprinkle the sunflower or sesame seeds and the yeast flakes, if using, over the top. Bake in the oven for 50 to 60 minutes, until bubbling and golden. Serve at once.

• Omit the cheese.

Couscous with Spicy Vegetables

Couscous consists of tiny pearls of pasta made from finely milled semolina wheat. It is widely used in North African countries, where it has given its name to this traditional dish served with a delicious vegetable stew. The only accompaniment it needs is a crisp green salad. Bulgur wheat may be substituted for the couscous. Serves 4 to 6

1⅓ cups chick-peas, soaked
4½ cups cold water
1¼ cups couscous
1¾ cups hot water
2 tablespoons olive oil
2 cups chopped white cabbage
1 teaspoon cayenne pepper
1 teaspoon paprika
2 teaspoons yellow mustard seeds
2 potatoes, diced

2 green bell peppers, cored, seeded, and diced
2⅔ cups thickly sliced zucchini
1¾ cups sliced okra
2 carrots, cut into thick slices
3 cups chopped tomatoes
⅓ cup raisins (optional)
Salt and pepper
2 tablespoons chopped fresh parsley
Parsley sprigs, to garnish

1 Drain the chick-peas and place in a pan with the cold water. Half cover and cook over medium heat for 1 to 1½ hours, until tender; drain and set aside to cool.

2 Put the couscous into a bowl, cover with the hot water, and leave to soak for 15 minutes. Meanwhile, heat the oil in a large pan, which a steamer will fit over. Add the cabbage to the pan and sauté lightly until softened. Stir in the spices and cook over medium heat for 1 minute. Add the potatoes and continue cooking for 3 to 4 minutes, until they begin to soften. Add the green bell peppers, zucchini, okra, carrots, tomatoes, cooked chick-peas, and raisins, if using.

3 Drain the couscous thoroughly and put into a steamer or colander lined with cheesecloth. Fit this over the pan of vegetables, making sure the bottom does not touch the vegetables. Place the lid on and steam the couscous for 20 minutes, stirring the vegetables occasionally until they are tender and the couscous is heated through. Season both the couscous and vegetables with salt and pepper to taste. Add the chopped parsley to the vegetables.

4 Transfer the couscous to a large, round serving dish and separate the grains with a fork. Pour the vegetables into a separate dish, or make a well in the mound of couscous and place the vegetables in it. Serve at once, garnished with parsley sprigs.

Barley One of the most ancient grains, barley has remained in the diet of many cultures around the world for a good reason. Its slightly sweet taste and chewy texture combine well with most vegetables and seasonings, especially in soups and casseroles. It is a highly nutritious food, rich in iron, calcium, potassium, B vitamins, and protein, as well as fiber. It has a cooling, anti-inflammatory effect on the body. Traditionally, barley water was fed to convalescents and used in cooling summer drinks. It is important to buy hulled barley, not the pearl barley available in supermarkets, which has has had the nutritious hull and bran layers removed. Barley is easy to cook using the same method as brown rice (see chart on page 46). It is especially tasty and healthy when preroasted; a very acid-forming grain, barley has an alkaline effect on the body when roasted. Roasted barley can be ground and sprinkled over cereals or used as a coffee substitute. Barley is also very good sprouted (when it is known as barley grass), providing a rich source of chlorophyll, beta-carotene, and minerals.

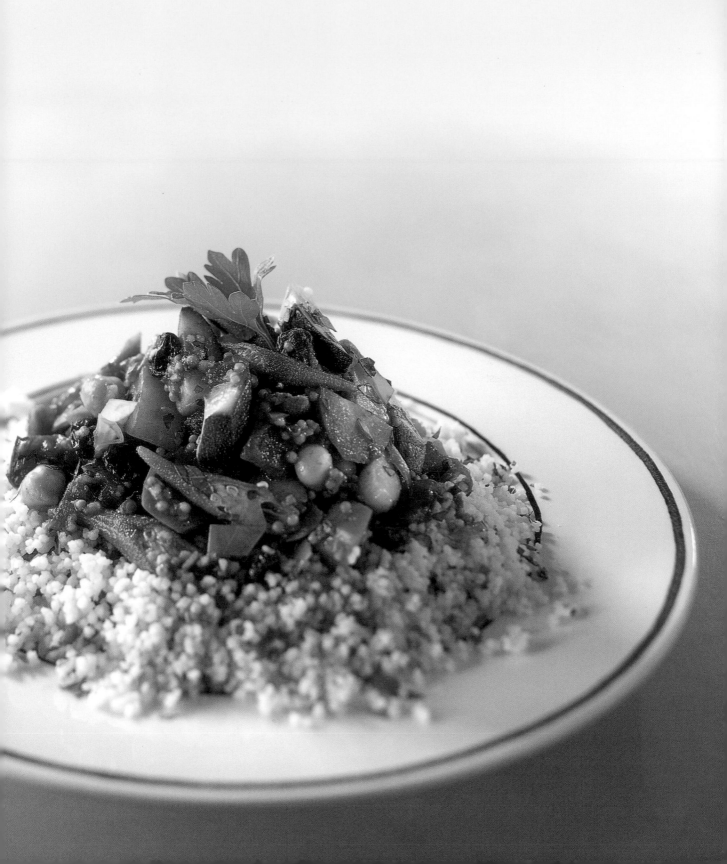

Creole Barley

This is barley with a bite, proving the point you do not need to spend a lot of money for well-balanced yet tasty food. Serves 6

1 tablespoon olive oil
2½ teaspoons cumin seeds
1 large red bell pepper, cored, seeded, and diced
2 sticks of celery, diced
¼ teaspoon crushed dried chilies
2 teaspoons dried oregano

3 tomatoes, diced
1½ cups hulled barley, rinsed
1 quart water
1 teaspoon salt
1 to 2 tablespoons chopped fresh cilantro

1 Heat the oil in a heavy pan and sauté the cumin seeds over high heat for a few seconds, taking care not to burn them. Add the red bell pepper, celery, dried chilies, and oregano and stir-fry for 2 minutes.

2 Add the diced tomatoes, barley, water, and salt. Bring to a boil, half cover, and simmer for 35 to 40 minutes, until the barley is tender and the liquid is absorbed. Add the chopped cilantro and serve at once.

Barley with Tomatoes, Olives, and Dill

This is a very elegant way of using barley, a hearty grain. Served with Ratatouille (page 89), this makes a delicious Mediterranean-style meal. An interesting variation is to omit the oil and dry roast the barley until it becomes aromatic, then add the water. This gives the dish a slightly smoky taste, and a more drying effect on the body. Serves 4 to 6

1 tablespoon oil
Generous 1 cup hulled barley, rinsed
2½ cups boiling water
3½ cups chopped tomatoes
½ cup pitted and finely chopped ripe olives

2 teaspoons dried dillweed
⅔ cup sour cream or drained ricotta cheese
Salt and pepper to taste
1 cup grated vegetarian cheese
4 ounces tomatoes, sliced

1 Heat the oil in a large pan and sauté the barley for 3 to 4 minutes. Add the boiling water and cook for 35 to 40 minutes, until tender. Meanwhile, heat the oven to 375°F.

2 Drain the barley. Combine all the ingredients, except for half the grated cheese and the sliced tomatoes, and spoon into a baking dish. Top with the remaining cheese and tomato slices.

3 Bake in the oven for 10 to 15 minutes, until the cheese melts and is beginning to brown. Serve at once.

• For a vegan version, use 7 ounces silken tofu instead of the sour cream or drained ricotta. Sprinkle with nutritional yeast flakes instead of cheese or omit entirely.
• For a vegetable-rich dish, sauté a selection of chopped vegetables, such as celery, red and green bell peppers, carrots, and zucchini, in a little butter or oil until soft and add to the mixture before baking.

Oats Renowned for their warming properties and used as a staple food in many cold climate cultures of the world, oats are high in fiber and rich in vitamin E, B vitamins, and the minerals calcium, potassium, and magnesium. They increase general vitality and are beneficial to the nervous system, helping to relieve stress and tension. Their high silicon content makes them desirable for healthy arterial walls and the renewal of all connective tissues. They are soothing to stomach and intestinal walls, and help to lower cholesterol. Rolled oats make a good thickening agent in soups, gravies, sauces, and stews. Old-fashioned rolled oats commonly available in health-food stores are preferable to the quick-cooking variety sold in supermarkets.

East-West Hot Pot *This crunchy hot pot makes an unusual lunch dish, and shows just how versatile oats are.* Serves 4 to 6

1 tablespoon oil
1¼ cups rolled oats
⅓ cup raw peanuts
⅔ cup peas or sliced green beans
Scant 1 cup chopped carrots
½ teaspoon cayenne pepper, or 4 or 5 green
    chilies, seeded and chopped

1 small tomato, chopped
1 teaspoon salt
1¾ cups boiling water
1 tablespoon grated vegetarian cheese (optional)
1 tablespoon butter or margarine
Coconut or Mint Chutney (page 125), to serve

1 Heat the oil in a heavy pan. Add the rolled oats and peanuts and sauté over medium heat for about 1 minute. Stir in the vegetables, cayenne or chilies, tomato, and salt. Add the boiling water, cover, and cook over medium heat for about 5 minutes, or until the vegetables are tender.

2 Remove the pan from the heat and add the grated cheese and butter or margarine. Serve with coconut or mint chutney.

Golden Oat Bake *Yoga has been defined as "balance of mind." This is a very harmonizing dish. Zucchini, like oats, have a calming effect on the nervous system. Served with Spiced Spring Carrots (page 84), this is a delicious, comforting dish for a cold winter's day.* Serves 6

3 tablespoons oil
Scant ½ cup chopped celery
2½ cups rolled oats
2⅓ cups grated zucchini
½ cup grated vegetarian cheese, or
    3 to 4 tablespoons nutritional yeast flakes and
    1 tablespoon margarine

2 tablespoons soy flour dissolved in
    2 tablespoons water
4 tablespoons wheat germ
⅔ cup sunflower seeds, toasted
¼ teaspoon freshly grated nutmeg
1 teaspoon salt

1 Heat the oven to 375°F. Heat the oil in a pan and sauté the celery over medium heat until soft. Stir in all the other ingredients and mix well.

2 Press the mixture into a well-greased 9- x 5-inch bread pan. Bake in the oven for 30 minutes. Turn out to serve.

• Replace the zucchini with 2 large carrots, grated. Substitute ½ teaspoon Italian seasoning and ½ teaspoon celery seeds for the sunflower seeds and nutmeg.

Millet For those with gluten allergies, millet is one of the few gluten-free grains. It is easy to digest, with a cooling and soothing effect on the digestive system. Millet is high in vitamins and minerals, especially iron, magnesium, and potassium, as well as fiber and silicon, and helps the body in repair, cleansing, and elimination. Millet can be cooked in two ways. Cooking it with plenty of water results in a thick consistency, ideal for stuffings, burgers, and toppings on vegetables. If toasted first and cooked with a little less water, the result is a fluffy grain similar to couscous.

Stovetop Millet Cakes

These cakes are like thick pancakes. They make a full meal when served with Tomato Sauce (page 123) or Salsa (page 124), steamed vegetables, and a mixed salad. Other vegetables may be substituted for the zucchini. The cakes can be reheated in a toaster. Serves 4 to 6

2 cups millet	1 teaspoon grated lemon zest
1 quart water	3 tablespoons whole wheat flour
Pinch of salt	2 tablespoons oil
1⅓ cups chopped zucchini	7 ounces firm tofu, crumbled

1 Place the millet in a large pan with the water and salt. Bring to a boil, cover, and simmer for about 30 minutes. Add the zucchini, bring back to a boil, and simmer for 10 minutes longer; leave to cool. When cold, mash the millet and zucchini. Add the remaining ingredients and stir to make a thick batter. Add a little extra water, if necessary.

2 Heat a lightly oiled, large skillet. Cook two or three cakes at a time; for each one, place a handful of millet mixture into the pan and press it down with a wet metal spatula. Cook over medium heat for 3 to 4 minutes on each side, until golden brown. Keep warm until they are all cooked.

Millet with Leafy Greens

Kale has 14 times more iron than red meat (gram for gram) and spinach has 11 times the amount, so this is an excellent dish for anyone worried about getting enough iron on a vegetarian diet. Serve with a salad and Spiced Spring Carrots (page 84) for a nutritious meal. Serves 6

4 tablespoons butter or margarine	1 tablespoon whole wheat flour
1½ cups millet	1 cup warm milk or soy milk
3⅓ cups boiling water	2 tablespoons grated vegetarian cheese or
Scant 1 cup finely chopped celery	nutritional yeast flakes
4½ cups finely shredded spinach and/or	Salt
young kale	Pinch of freshly grated nutmeg

1 Melt half the butter or margarine in a pan and sauté the millet over medium heat for about 5 minutes, stirring. Add the boiling water and cook gently for about 20 minutes, or until the millet is tender and all the water is absorbed; set aside.

2 Melt the remaining butter or margarine in a separate pan and sauté the celery for 5 to 10 minutes, until soft. Stir in the spinach and/or kale and cook for a few minutes until wilted. Stir in the flour and add the warm milk, stirring to prevent lumps forming. Reduce the heat and cook for a few minutes. Stir in the millet and cheese or yeast flakes and season with salt and nutmeg. Mix well and serve.

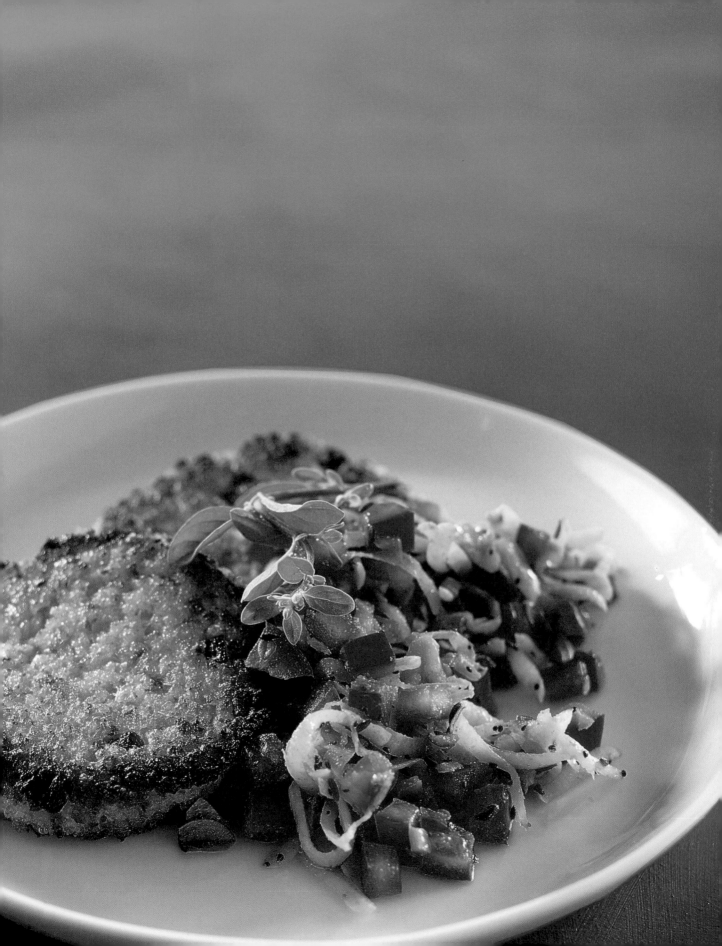

Buckwheat A staple of the Eastern European diet, buckwheat is a power-packed grain containing all eight essential amino acids. It is also rich in the B vitamins, vitamin E, and the bioflavonoid rutin, which aids circulatory problems. A rich source of fiber and silica, buckwheat has a warming and drying effect on the body. It is astringent with very alkaline properties.

Buckwheat is fast cooking, so it is a boon to anyone with a hectic lifestyle. It can be bought either roasted (known as kasha) or unroasted. Roasted buckwheat has a richer flavor. It can be used like rice, served in stews, and with vegetables. Cooked until soft, it can be molded into shapes and baked. Buckwheat flour is frequently used in Oriental cooking to make pancakes and noodles.

Buckwheat Burgers

Every summer we have a kids camp at our ashram in Canada. The children meditate, do asanas, and practice Karma Yoga, as well as going swimming and hiking. They work up a healthy appetite and these burgers are perfectly suited for kid-sized appetites—for kids of all ages. Serve them with any sauce (pages 122 to 125) or on a bun. Serves 6

1 cup unroasted buckwheat groats
1¾ cups hot water
1 or 2 carrots, finely diced
½ ounce dulse seaweed, soaked in enough water to cover for 5 minutes, then chopped

Generous 2 cups rolled oats
3 tablespoons tamari
A little wheat, rye, or rice flour
Oil for brushing
Sesame seeds (optional)

1 Toast the buckwheat groats gently for a few minutes in a dry, heavy pan. When the grain starts to turn brown, add the hot water. Cover and cook for about 15 minutes. Meanwhile, heat the oven to 400°F.

2 Remove the pan from the heat and stir in the carrots, dulse, rolled oats, and tamari; mix well. Form the mixture into burgers. Spread the flour out on a flat plate and coat each burger, shaking to remove any excess flour. Place the burgers on a lightly greased baking sheet. Brush the tops with a little oil and sprinkle with sesame seeds, if using. Bake in the oven for about 20 minutes, until brown. Serve at once.

Kasha Varnishkas

An Eastern European specialty, this recipe was one of Swami Saradananda's childhood favorites. Serves 4 to 6

4 ounces dried farfalle (butterfly-shaped) pasta
½ cup roasted buckwheat
3⅓ cups boiling water
1 teaspoon salt

4 tablespoons butter or margarine
Rich Brown Gravy with Vegetables (page 122), to serve

1 Cook the pasta in a large pan of boiling water until tender; drain and set aside. Meanwhile, toast the buckwheat in a dry, heavy pan over low heat for a few minutes, stirring constantly. When the grain starts to turn brown, slowly add the boiling water, stirring constantly. Cover and cook over low heat for 10 to 15 minutes, until tender.

2 Remove the buckwheat from the heat and mix with the salt and butter or margarine. Drain the pasta and add to the buckwheat. Serve hot with the gravy.

Japanese Buckwheat Noodles
Soba noodles, as buckwheat noodles are known in Japan, are a delight for those on a gluten-free diet who are missing the joys of pasta. Serves 4 to 6

9 ounces buckwheat noodles
3-inch piece of kombu seaweed
2½ cups shredded cabbage, or 7 ounces watercress
⅔ cup peas or corn kernels

1 carrot, chopped
4½ cups water
2 to 3 tablespoons tamari
Toasted nori seaweed, to garnish (optional)

1 Cook the noodles in a large pan of boiling water; drain, rinse, and set aside.

2 Wipe the kombu with a damp cloth to remove the excess salt, then place it in a pan with the vegetables and water and bring to a boil. Reduce the heat, cover, and simmer for 5 minutes.

3 Discard the kombu and add the cooked noodles and tamari to the vegetables. Heat slowly for about 2 minutes to warm the cooked noodles through again. Serve at once, garnished with a little toasted nori, if desired.

• Use whole wheat spaghetti instead of the buckwheat noodles.

Buckwheat Salad with Arame
Arame is a very mild-tasting seaweed, rich in potassium and calcium. Combined with buckwheat, it makes a lovely salad. You can make a cool version of this piquant salad using cucumber, or a crunchy version using sunflower seeds. Serves 4 to 6

½ cup roasted buckwheat
1¾ cups plus 2 tablespoons water
2 tablespoons oil
1 tablespoon lemon juice
1 to 2 tablespoons tamari
¾-inch piece of fresh gingerroot, peeled and grated

¼ teaspoon pepper
1 to 2 tablespoons arame, soaked in enough water to cover for 10 minutes
1 cup carrots, cut into matchsticks
¼ of a cucumber, cut into matchsticks, or 1 to 2 tablespoons sunflower seeds, toasted
1 tablespoon chopped fresh parsley

1 Place the buckwheat and water in a heavy pan and bring to a boil. Reduce the heat, cover the pan, and simmer very slowly for 15 minutes, until all the water is absorbed and the buckwheat is tender; leave to cool.

2 Combine the oil, lemon juice, tamari, ginger, and pepper to make a dressing.

3 Cut the arame into 2-inch pieces and mix it into the cooled buckwheat with the carrots, cucumber or sunflower seeds, and the lemon and ginger dressing. Garnish with the chopped parsley and serve at once.

Corn Alternatively considered to be a grain and a vegetable, corn has a tonic effect on the body. It is gluten-free, helps build bones and muscles, is excellent for the nervous system and brain, and may help to lower the risk of heart disease. Corn is available as corn cobs, kernels, cornmeal (also sold as maizemeal in some countries), cornstarch, and polenta. Cornmeal can be made into porridge or used in baking. As cornmeal has a high percentage of oil, it does not keep well, so it is best to buy small quantities and use it up quickly. In parts of India, cornmeal is a staple ingredient in the rotis, or flat breads, that are prepared fresh at every meal. It is also used to thicken curries and added to batters and vegetable dishes. Cornstarch is finely ground cornmeal used mainly as a thickening agent. Polenta is dried and ground corn, similar to cornmeal but with a slightly more granular texture. It is made into a porridge which can be eaten hot or left to cool, sliced and broiled.

Herbed Polenta with Fresh Corn
Polenta is a specialty of northern Italy. In this recipe, fresh corn enhances the taste of the polenta, while the rosemary adds a vibrancy to the dish. Rosemary was considered a sacred plant in ancient Greece and Rome. It is claimed to have a profound effect on the cleansing and energizing of the liver, and to improve the memory, and lift depression.
Serves 4 to 6

1 ear of corn	2 teaspoons finely chopped fresh rosemary
Scant 1½ cups cornmeal	2 tablespoons olive oil
3⅓ cups water	Tomato Sauce (page 123) or Ratatouille
1 teaspoon salt	(page 89), to serve

1 Cook the corn on the cob in boiling water for 8 to 10 minutes, until tender. Using a sharp knife, remove the kernels; set aside.

2 Stir the cornmeal into 1 cup of the water to make a batter. In a large, heavy pan, bring the remaining water and salt to a boil. Add the cornmeal batter all at once and stir continuously until the batter is well blended. Add the chopped rosemary.

3 Reduce the heat so the batter simmers and stir constantly for 10 to 15 minutes, until the polenta pulls away from the side of the pan. Stir in the cooked corn kernels.

4 Pour the polenta into a 10-inch pie plate, smooth the top with a metal spatula, and leave it to cool. Once set, cut the polenta into slices and fry in a little olive oil, until slightly crisp. Alternatively, brush with oil and bake or broil. Serve with tomato sauce or ratatouille.

• Serve the polenta in slices without frying or baking it.
• For extra richness and flavor, stir in 1 tablespoon olive oil while the polenta is cooking.
• Stir 2 tablespoons grated vegetarian cheese into the polenta at the end of cooking.
• For a more complex flavor, omit the salt and blend in a little light miso when the polenta is cooked.

Cornbread

Cornmeal gives bread a golden color as well as an appetizing nutty flavor and crisp texture. Use finely ground whole wheat flour (called whole wheat pastry flour), which is available from health-food stores. You can vary the proportion of cornmeal and wheat flour for different tastes and consistencies. Serves 8 to 10

3¼ cups cornmeal
1⅔ cups whole wheat pastry flour
1 tablespoon baking powder
1 teaspoon salt
⅔ cup oil

7½ tablespoons maple syrup, honey, or barley malt syrup
About 1½ cups milk or soy milk
2 tablespoons plain yogurt (optional)

1 Heat the oven to 375°F. Combine all the dry ingredients in a bowl. In a separate bowl, mix the wet ingredients together.

2 Mix the wet ingredients into the dry ones to make a thick, pourable batter, stirring well; if it is too thick, add more milk. Transfer to a greased 8-inch square cake pan and bake in the oven for 35 to 40 minutes.

• Replace 1¼ cups of the cornmeal with 1¾ cups bran flakes.
• Make 24 small or 12 large corn muffins. Spoon the batter into muffin pans and bake at 375°F for 15 to 20 minutes for small muffins, 20 to 25 minutes for large.

Corn Fritters

Too much fried food is not good, but occasionally the tongue may be gratified with a few of these tasty tidbits. Corn fritters are a traditional Bahamian dish, and they can be served with any chutney. Special thanks to Jyoti for this recipe. Makes 24 to 30 small fritters

1½ cups whole wheat flour
½ cup chick-pea (besan) flour
2¼ cups fresh corn kernels (cut off the cobs) or canned corn, drained
4 to 6 fresh green chilies
½ teaspoon turmeric
1 teaspoon salt
¼ teaspoon pepper

Juice of 1 lemon
1-inch piece of fresh gingerroot, peeled and grated
1 bunch of fresh cilantro or parsley, finely chopped
3 tablespoons oil, plus oil for deep-frying
2 tablespoons plain yogurt
½ teaspoon baking soda

1 Mix all the ingredients, except the oil, yogurt, and baking soda, in a heatproof bowl.

2 Heat the 3 tablespoons of oil and when it is very hot pour it over the mixture in the bowl and fold in.

3 In a separate bowl, combine the yogurt and baking soda. Add it to the corn to bind the batter.

4 Heat the oil for frying. Form the batter into little balls (about ½ tablespoon at a time) and deep-fry a few at a time in the hot oil for 1 to 2 minutes, turning them with a slotted spoon. Transfer to paper towels to drain.

• Any vegetable may be substituted for, or added to, the corn. Chop the vegetable(s) into small pieces. Apples, pears, or bananas with grated fresh coconut can also be substituted.
• Add cheese or tofu to the fritter batter, either by themselves or with fruit or vegetables.

PROTEIN
PRANA

*" The foods which contain protein should not be more
than one-fourth the weight of the amount of vegetables
and fruit taken at a meal. Do not eat too much protein.
An excess of protein overtaxes the liver and the
kidneys and causes serious diseases."*

Swami Sivananda

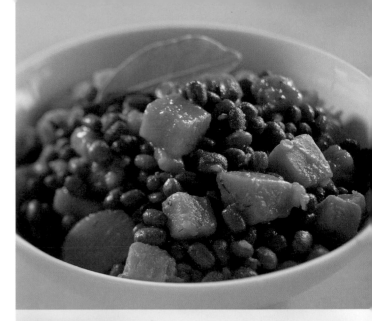

"Prana," often translated as "life force" or "vital energy" may be more accurately described as the energy that produces this physical manifestation. Our bodies are completely regulated by the force of prana. Each cell is controlled and built as much by prana as by protein.

To quote the Swami Vishnu-devananda in *The Complete Illustrated Book of Yoga*: "Prana is in the air, but is not the oxygen, nor any of its chemical constituents. It is in the food, water, and in the sunlight, yet it is not vitamin, heat, or light-rays. Food, water and air are only the media through which the prana is carried. We absorb this prana through the food we eat, the water we drink, and the air we breathe."

Food that is fresh and pure by nature is full of prana. When it is prepared with loving attention, that prana is enhanced. But if the cook is upset while cooking, the prana will be drained from the food and it won't satisfy your needs—spiritual, mental, or physical.

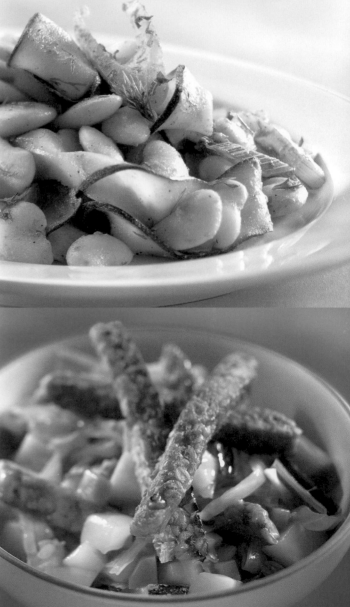

Protein supplies the physical materials for growth and the repair of cells and tissues; as the body requires continual overhauling and renewal, a constant supply of protein is needed. Proteins are formed by the linkage of 22 different "building blocks" called amino acids. The value of protein depends on its amino-acid content. The difference between proteins is due to the number, arrangement, and proportion of the different amino acids.

Legumes (beans) are the most common sources of vegetarian protein, but nuts, seeds, and cheese are also excellent. Legumes combined with grains form the basics of a vegetarian diet. Legumes are low in fat, high in fiber, and rich in iron, B vitamins, and trace minerals. Whereas many plants rob the soil of vital nutrients as they grow, legumes take nitrogen from the atmosphere and restore it in large amounts to the soil. By nourishing your body with legumes, you also help to nourish the planet.

In yoga, everything is best done gradually and in moderation. If you are adding legumes to your diet, start slowly, as it might take your system a while to get used to their gas-producing propensity. Adzuki beans, lentils, mung beans, and split peas are the easiest to digest and may be eaten on a daily basis. They may be sprouted and eaten raw. Other legumes need cooking even when sprouted, and should be eaten no more than once or twice a week.

Most legumes need soaking before cooking; rinse thoroughly and pick out husks, stones, or dirt, then soak in enough water to cover. After the appropriate time, drain, place the legumes in a large pan and add fresh water (the amount varies from twice the volume to four times the volume, see chart). Don't add salt, as this toughens legumes; use a little seaweed (such as kombu), if you like. Bring to a boil: if cooking adzuki, black, black-eyed, or kidney beans, boil vigorously for 10 minutes; if soybeans boil for 1 hour. Skim off any foam, then half cover the pan, and simmer the legumes for the appropriate cooking time (see below), until soft but not mushy. About 1½ cups dried beans will feed four to six people.

COOKING LEGUMES

Legume	Soaking time	Volume of water	Cooking time
Adzuki beans	3 to 4 hours	2 to 3 times	45 to 60 minutes
Black beans	3 to 4 hours	2 to 3 times	1 hour
Black-eyed beans	1 to 2 hours	3 times	45 minutes
Butter beans	8 to 12 hours	2 to 3 times	1 to 1½ hours
Canellini beans	4 to 8 hours	3 times	1 to 1½ hours
Chick-peas	8 to 12 hours	4 times	1 to 1½ hours
Fava beans	8 to 12 hours	4 times	1 hour
Kidney beans	8 to 10 hours	2 to 3 times	1 to 1½ hours
Lentils (green or brown)	Not required	3 times	30 to 40 minutes
Lentils, Puy	Not required	Twice	25 to 35 minutes
Lentils, Red	Not required	Twice	15 to 30 minutes
Mung beans	Not required	3 to 4 times	30 to 45 minutes
Pinto beans	8 to 12 hours	3 to 4 times	1 to 1½ hours
Soybeans	8 to 12 hours	4 times	2 to 4 hours
Split peas	Not required	3 times	35 to 45 minutes

Kitcheree

People love kitcheree! This hearty, one-pot dish is widely eaten in India, especially by sadhus, who leave it to cook while they are meditating. During the Sivananda Sadhana intensive course for our yoga teachers, we serve it daily. If you are doing a lot of pranayama or live in a cold climate, be sure to add the ghee. Kitcheree gives strength and vitality, and is often used as part of a body detox program, after kriyas (cleansing exercises) and upon breaking of a fast. In Ayurveda, kitcheree often plays a key role in nutritional healing. Serves 4 to 6

1¼ cups mung beans
1¼ cups basmati rice
1 tablespoon oil
1 teaspoon brown mustard seeds
1 teaspoon cumin seeds

2 sticks of celery, finely chopped
1 teaspoon ground coriander
Salt
2 tablespoons ghee (optional)

1 Place the mung beans in a pan with three to four times their volume of water. Bring to a boil, lower the heat, cover, and simmer for 30 to 45 minutes, until tender. Meanwhile, cook the rice separately. Set both aside.

2 Heat the oil in a wok or pan. Add the mustard and cumin seeds and cook over high heat until they "pop."

3 Add the celery and sauté over medium heat for about 5 minutes. Stir in the ground coriander, cooked rice, and mung beans. Cook for another 10 minutes, stirring. Season to taste with salt. Add the ghee, if using, and serve at once.

• Brown rice or barley may be substituted for the basmati rice. They both make the dish even heartier. Another popular variation at our ashram in Canada is to use presoaked hijiki (seaweed) instead of the celery.

Swami Gayatri's Mung Beans

The popular standby of our 70-year-young grandmother, who has taught so many people to cook and to serve with love. Serves 4

1 cup mung beans
3 cups water
1 cup unpacked unsweetened dried coconut
2 tablespoons oil
1 teaspoon black mustard seeds

5 or 6 curry leaves (page 156)
¼ teaspoon turmeric
1 teaspoon salt
1 heaped teaspoon ground cumin
1 teaspoon ground fennel (optional)

1 Place the mung beans in a pan with the water. Bring to a boil, lower the heat, cover, and simmer for 30 to 45 minutes, until the beans are soft. Meanwhile, soak the coconut in a bowl with enough warm water to cover, about ¼ cup.

2 Heat the oil in a heavy skillet. Add the mustard seeds and cook over high heat until they "pop." Squeeze any water from the soaked coconut and add the coconut to the pan. Sauté for 2 to 3 minutes. Add the curry leaves, turmeric, and salt and stir well for about 1 minute.

3 Drain off any excess water from the mung beans and add them to the mixture. Stir over low heat for 2 minutes, then stir in the ground cumin and fennel. Transfer to a serving dish to serve.

White Beans with Zucchini and Herbs

White beans delicately flavored with curry powder and fennel are complemented by crisp ribbons of zucchini. Serves 4 to 6

2½ cups dried butter or fava beans, soaked
4½ cups water
2 tablespoons butter or margarine
1 tablespoon curry powder
1 large fennel head, chopped
2 tablespoons olive oil

Juice of ½ lemon
Salt and pepper
1 zucchini
3 tablespoons chopped fresh parsley
3 tablespoons chopped fresh dill

1 Drain the beans, place them in a pan, and cover with the water. Bring to a boil. Reduce the heat, cover, and simmer for 1 to 1½ hours, until tender.

2 Melt half of the butter or margarine in a large pan, stir in the curry powder and sauté the fennel over medium heat until it is translucent. Drain the beans and add them. Cover and cook over very low heat for 10 minutes. Season the beans with the olive oil, lemon juice, and salt and pepper to taste. Transfer to a serving dish.

3 Cut the zucchini lengthwise into long ribbons. Melt the remaining butter or margarine in a skillet. Add the zucchini ribbons, chopped parsley, and dill and sauté slowly over medium heat, stirring frequently, until some of the zucchini ribbons are lightly touched with brown; they should soften slightly but still keep some of their "bite"—take care not to break them. Use to garnish the beans and serve immediately.

Kamala's Pilaf *Kamala runs an affiliated Sivananda Yoga Centre in the Blue Mountains of Australia; this is one of the favorite recipes for after-satsang (group meditation) supper.* Serves 4 to 6

½ cup yellow split peas
½ cup millet
2 tablespoons ghee or oil
2 x 2-inch cinnamon sticks, broken in half
½ teaspoon turmeric
½ teaspoon garam masala
1 teaspoon salt
½ teaspoon cayenne pepper (optional)

1 teaspoon ground cumin
2 tomatoes, chopped
4½ cups boiling water
2 tablespoons oil
½ teaspoon black mustard seeds
4½ cups chopped fresh spinach,
    stems removed

1 Rinse and soak the split peas for about 2 hours; drain well and set aside. Dry toast the millet for 5 minutes, remove from the heat, and set aside. Heat the ghee or oil in a heavy skillet. Add the cinnamon sticks, turmeric, and garam masala and sauté for 8 to 10 minutes over low heat. Stir in the split peas, toasted millet, salt, and cayenne pepper, if using. Sauté the mixture for 8 to 10 minutes longer.

2 Add the ground cumin and chopped tomatoes, stir well, and cook for 3 to 4 minutes. Add the boiling water and simmer for 30 to 35 minutes, stirring occasionally. About 10 minutes before the lentils are cooked, heat the oil in a separate skillet. Add the mustard seeds and toast until they "pop." Add the chopped spinach, mix thoroughly, cover, and simmer for 5 minutes. Add the spinach and spice mixture to the cooked split pea mixture, cover, and cook over low heat for 5 minutes longer, stirring occasionally.

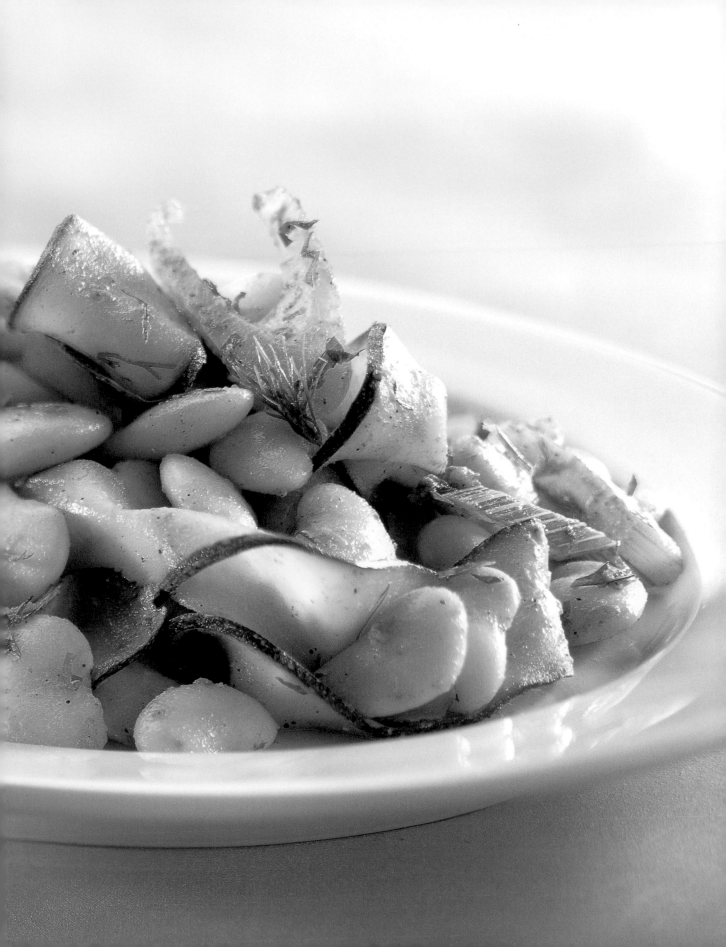

Swami Saradananda's Baked Beans

This is a traditional New England-style, slow-cooking dish—put it in the oven in the morning and forget about it until almost dinnertime, apart from checking it from time to time. Navy or pinto beans may be substituted to equally satisfy nutritional needs and hungry appetites. Serve with Cornbread (page 65) or rice. Serves 6

1 cup dried kidney beans, soaked
3½ cups hot water
2 bay leaves, crumbled
7½ tablespoons molasses
1 teaspoon mustard powder

10 black peppercorns, crushed slightly
4 tablespoons tomato paste
1 potato, chopped
1 carrot, grated
1 teaspoon salt

1 Heat the oven to 275°F. Drain the beans and place in a pan with the hot water. Bring to a boil and boil vigorously for 10 minutes. Skim off the white foam. Transfer the beans and cooking water to a baking dish.

2 Add the bay leaves, molasses, mustard powder, and peppercorns. Cover the dish with a tight-fitting lid and bake for 6 to 8 hours, checking occasionally to make sure there is enough water.

3 Stir in the tomato paste, potato, carrot, and salt. Increase the oven temperature to 300°F and bake for 2 hours longer; serve hot.

• After cooking, turn off the oven and leave the covered baking dish inside overnight for "Beans on Toast" in the morning.

Prema and Dattatreya's Cinnamon Beans

Dattatreya, a 73-year-young yogi who can still put both legs behind his head, is a native of Italy. Now teaching yoga in London, he and his wife Prema have adapted this Italian dish. It is always a favorite at our Christmas party, and is especially nice served with Herbed Polenta with Fresh Corn (page 64). Serves 4

1½ cups black-eyed peas, soaked
14 ounces tomatoes
4 tablespoons olive oil
1-inch piece of fresh gingerroot, peeled and
  grated

4 sticks of celery, finely chopped
1 cup water
2 teaspoons tomato paste
2 teaspoons ground cinnamon
Salt and pepper to taste

1 Drain the beans, place them in a pan, and cover with fresh water. Bring to a boil and boil vigorously for 10 minutes. Half cover and simmer for 45 minutes, until tender.

2 Meanwhile, scald, skin, and chop the tomatoes.

3 Heat the oil in a pan over low heat. Add the ginger and celery and fry for 2 to 3 minutes. Drain the beans and add to the pan with the water, tomato paste, cinnamon, and salt and pepper. Stir and cook for 15 minutes longer. Add the tomatoes and cook for 5 minutes longer. Serve at once.

Chili con Veggies *A tasty dish that can assist in making the*
changes in diet (and lifestyle) gradually, as is usually best in the long term. Even non-
vegetarian friends will love this served with Cornbread (page 65). Vary the dish
sometimes by using black beans instead of kidney beans. Serves 4 to 6

1 cup kidney beans, soaked
4 tablespoons oil
1½ teaspoons chili powder
½ teaspoon ground cumin
½ teaspoon turmeric
1 large green bell pepper, cored, seeded,
  and chopped

3 sticks of celery, chopped
1 large carrot, chopped
2 large tomatoes, chopped
4 tablespoons tomato paste
2 to 3 tablespoons lemon juice (optional)
Salt to taste

1 Drain the kidney beans, place them in a pan, and cover with fresh water. Bring to a boil and boil vigorously for 10 minutes. Half cover and simmer gently for 1 to 1½ hours longer, until the beans are tender; drain and set aside.

2 Heat the oil in a heavy skillet and sauté the spices for a few minutes. Add the green bell pepper, celery, and carrot and cook for 4 to 5 minutes, until the vegetables are slightly soft. Stir in the tomatoes and tomato paste and simmer for 15 minutes. Add the cooked beans and simmer for 15 minutes longer. Season with lemon juice and salt and serve at once.

Spanish-Style Chick-Peas *Chick-peas are best eaten as*
a midday meal. When served as the evening meal they tend to make getting up for
morning meditation more difficult. Serves 4 to 6

Generous 1 cup chick-peas, soaked
3 tablespoons olive oil
Pinch of ground coriander
Pinch of ground ginger
Pinch of freshly grated nutmeg
1 green bell pepper, cored, seeded, and chopped

1 red bell pepper, cored, seeded, and chopped
1 fresh green chili, seeded and chopped
  (optional)
1 pound tomatoes, chopped
1 teaspoon salt
¼ teaspoon pepper

1 Drain the chick-peas, place in a pan, and cover with fresh water. Add 1 tablespoon of the olive oil. Bring to a boil, half cover and simmer for 1 to 1½ hours, until the chick-peas are tender; drain and set aside.

2 Heat the remaining oil in a heavy skillet. Add the spices, bell peppers, green chili, if using, and tomatoes and sauté until the vegetables are tender. Add the chick-peas, mix well, then cook together for about 2 minutes. Season with the salt and pepper and serve at once.

Adzuki Bean Stew
Adzuki beans are used extensively in Japanese cooking. This is a classic macrobiotic dish, best served on rice or millet. Serves 4 to 6

1 cup dried adzuki beans, soaked
2 bay leaves (optional)
4 cups water
2 cups peeled, seeded, and diced acorn or butternut squash

1 carrot, cubed or sliced
½ teaspoon dried thyme
1 teaspoon dried savory (optional)
2 to 4 tablespoons miso

1 Drain the beans and place in a pan with the bay leaves and water. Cook over medium heat for about 40 minutes, until almost tender, adding a little more water if necessary.

2 Add the squash, carrot, thyme, and savory, if using. Continue to simmer for about 20 minutes, until everything is tender, stirring occasionally; the stew should have a slightly dry consistency. Remove the pan from the heat and stir in the miso. Serve at once.

• Omit the bay leaves and add ½ ounce soaked hijiki at the same time as the vegetables.

Tamale-Bean Pie
This tasty Mexican pie is soft so it needs to be spooned rather than sliced. Serve with a green salad. Serves 4 to 6

Generous 1 cup dried pinto beans, soaked
3⅓ cups water
2 tablespoons oil
1 teaspoon black mustard seeds
2 teaspoons cumin seeds
1 large green bell pepper, cored, seeded, and chopped
2 to 3 fresh green chilies, seeded and chopped
4 tomatoes, chopped

1 teaspoon cayenne pepper
1 teaspoon dried oregano
½ to 1 teaspoon salt
Crust:
2 cups cornmeal
1 cup cold water
1 teaspoon salt
3⅓ cups boiling water

1 Drain the beans, place them in a pan, and cover with the water. Cook over medium heat, half covered, for 1 to 1½ hours, until tender; set aside.

2 Heat the oil in a large skillet. Add the mustard and cumin seeds and toast over high heat until they "pop." Add the green bell pepper and chilies and sauté until slightly soft. Stir in the tomatoes, cayenne pepper, and oregano and cook until the tomatoes are soft. Add the salt and pinto beans. Cook over low heat for about 10 minutes, stirring occasionally; set aside.

3 To make the crust, combine the cornmeal, cold water, and salt in a nonstick pan, stirring well. Place over medium heat, add the boiling water, and stir until smooth. Continue cooking for about 15 minutes, stirring occasionally. Meanwhile, heat the oven to 350°F.

4 Oil a baking dish or large, round pie plate and spread half of the cornmeal mixture on the bottom and around the sides to form a shell. Spoon the bean mixture into the shell and top with the remaining cornmeal. Cover the dish or pie plate with a lid or foil and bake in the oven for about 30 minutes. Serve hot.

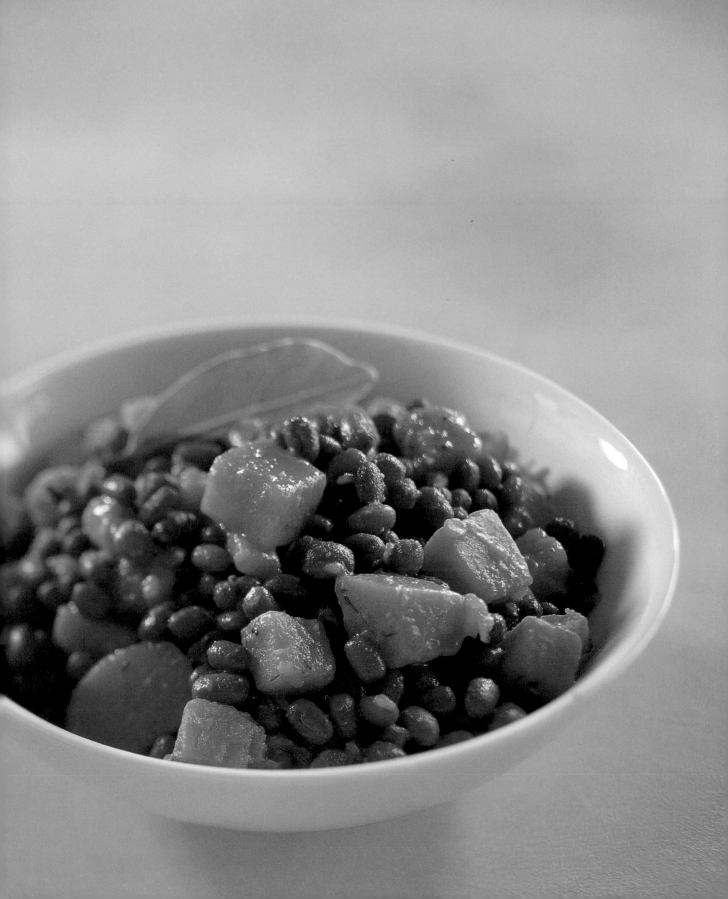

Lentil Dal
Often mistaken for a soup, dal is served over rice and/or with chapatis as the standard meal of northern India. For a simple meal, serve it with plain rice, yogurt, and Curried Vegetables (page 88). For a larger spread, add Rice Pilau (page 47), raita, and Chapatis (page 53). For a more aromatic dal, add a cinnamon stick and/or 5 or 6 cloves to the lentils while cooking. Serves 4 to 6

1 cup red lentils
3⅓ cups water
1 teaspoon turmeric
1 bay leaf
1 to 2 tablespoons ghee, butter, or oil
1 teaspoon mustard seeds

1 teaspoon cumin or fennel seeds
2 teaspoons ground coriander
2 tomatoes, coarsely chopped
1 teaspoon salt
½ to 1 tablespoon lemon juice (optional)
4 tablespoons chopped fresh cilantro

1 Place the lentils in a pan with the water, turmeric, and bay leaf. Simmer for 15 to 20 minutes, until the lentils are tender.

2 Meanwhile, heat the ghee, butter, or oil in a heavy skillet. Add the mustard and cumin or fennel seeds and cook over high heat until they "pop."

3 Add the ground coriander and tomatoes and cook for 5 minutes longer, then add the mixture to the cooked lentils. Add more water if the mixture is too thick, or cook a little longer to make it thicker. Add the salt and lemon juice, if desired. Stir in the chopped cilantro and serve at once.

Carrot-Cashew Slice
Carrots are renowned for strengthening the eyesight, celery for its calming effect on the nerves, and cabbage for its all-round healing properties. Serve with a simple boiled grain and a green salad. Topped with Tomato Sauce (page 123), this becomes a festive meal. Serves 4 to 6

1¼ cups millet
2½ cups water
1⅔ cups cashew nuts
2 tablespoons oil
4 carrots, grated
½ white cabbage, finely chopped

4 sticks of celery, finely sliced
1 tablespoon Italian seasoning
½ teaspoon freshly grated nutmeg
1 tablespoon tamari
Pinch of pepper

1 Place the millet in a large pan with the water. Simmer for 30 to 40 minutes, until tender.

2 Heat a dry skillet and toast the cashews over high heat for about 5 minutes, until lightly brown; set aside.

3 Meanwhile, heat the oven to 425°F.

4 Heat the oil in a pan. Add the vegetables and sauté over medium heat for about 15 minutes, until the vegetables are soft.

5 Add the cooked millet, toasted cashews, Italian seasoning, nutmeg, tamari, and pepper and mix well. Spoon into a greased 8½- x 4½-inch bread pan and bake in the oven for 15 minutes.

6 Leave to cool, then turn out of the pan. Cut into slices and serve.

Vegetable Pâté
Developed by Uma at the Sivananda Yoga Retreat in Nassau, this recipe is a favorite which has been passed from center to center. It is best cooked in advance and allowed to chill for a few hours. Serves 6 to 8

1 cup plus 4 tablespoons sunflower seeds
²/₃ cup whole wheat flour
½ ounce nutritional yeast flakes
2 tablespoons lemon juice
2 tablespoons butter or margarine
2 carrots
1 potato
1 stick of celery

Pinch of dried sage
1½ teaspoons dried thyme
1½ teaspoons dried basil or a bunch of fresh basil
1 teaspoon salt
1 cup warm water
Dash of pepper

1 Heat the oven to 400°F. Put all the ingredients into a food processor and blend for about ·4 minutes, until smooth. Alternatively, grate all the vegetables, grind the seeds in a blender, and mix everything together in a bowl.

2 Spoon the vegetable mixture into a greased 8½- x 4½-inch bread pan and bake in the oven for 1 hour. Leave to cool, then chill it in the refrigerator before serving. The pâté rises while cooking, but sinks as it cools.

• Substitute almonds, walnuts, or a mixture, for the sunflower seeds.

Sunflower-Sesame Rissoles
After Christmas at our center in London we have a Beginners' Week. After a few days of ashram life, the experienced "Karma Yogis" prepare the New Year's Eve feast. This party recipe was made by Gloria MacDonald. It is very nice served with Tomato Sauce (page 123) or Rich Brown Gravy (page 122). Serves 4 to 6

1½ cups sesame seeds
2²/₃ cups sunflower seeds
½ teaspoon dried marjoram
½ teaspoon dried oregano
½ teaspoon dried thyme
½ teaspoon dried basil
1 teaspoon ground cumin

1 tablespoon tamari
1 large green bell pepper, cored, seeded, and finely chopped
1 to 2 sticks of celery, finely chopped
1 carrot, grated
1 tomato, quartered

1 Heat the oven to 350°F. Grind the sesame seeds in a blender, then the sunflower seeds, making sure both seeds are not too finely ground because the rissoles need some texture. Put the seeds in a large bowl.

2 Stir in the herbs, cumin, and tamari, then the green bell pepper, celery, and carrot. Put the tomato into the blender and blend briefly, allowing small lumps to remain. Carefully stir the tomato into the seed mixture.

3 Take a handful of the mixture, form it into a smooth ball, and flatten it. Place it on a greased baking sheet. Repeat to make 12 to 16 rissoles. Bake the rissoles in the oven for 30 to 45 minutes, until brown.

• Make smaller rissoles and serve them as party food with dips.

Tempeh This is a soy food sold in densely packed cakes. Originating from Indonesia, tempeh has a stronger flavor than tofu, making it ideal for casseroles and stews, and it has a high protein and vitamin B12 content. It is sold chilled or frozen. Different varieties are made by combining soybeans with wheat, rice, millet, peanuts, and/or coconut. Like its cousin tofu, it is very versatile and can be baked, fried, marinated, and steamed. It can be pan-fried with herbs or spices and tossed into pasta, or added to grain dishes at the last moment. Highly nutritious, tempeh can be of benefit to frail people. Do not eat it raw; it needs to be thoroughly cooked.

Tempeh Stew *Serve this stew in bowls with cooked rice or barley or large chunks of fresh bread.* Serves 6

1 carrot, cubed or thinly sliced
1 turnip, cubed or thinly sliced
3/4 rutabaga, cubed
1/2 small cabbage, shredded
1 large zucchini or squash, cubed
1 strip of kombu seaweed, cut into
  small pieces

1 tablespoon fresh gingerroot, peeled
  and grated
1 3/4 cups water
1 to 2 tablespoons arrowroot
2 tablespoons oil
9 1/2 ounces tempeh, cut into thick strips
Tamari

1 Put the vegetables, kombu, ginger, and 1 1/4 cups of the water into a heavy pan, half cover, and simmer for about 10 minutes, until the vegetables are half cooked.

2 Put the remaining water in a small bowl and blend in 1 tablespoon arrowroot until it is smooth. Stir this into the stew and continue stirring until it thickens. (If it comes back to the boil and has not thickened, repeat the process.) Continue cooking until all the vegetables are tender. Meanwhile, heat the oil in a separate pan and sauté the tempeh until golden brown. Add it to the stew just before serving. Season to taste with tamari.

Tempeh with Sesame Seeds *This light dish can be served with a simple grain. Tofu can be substituted for the tempeh.* Serves 3 to 4

8 ounces tempeh, cut into strips
2 tablespoons olive oil or dark sesame oil
2 to 3 tablespoon sesame seeds
Sauce:
1 tablespoon oil
3 to 4 tomatoes, chopped

2 teaspoons grated fresh gingerroot
2 tablespoons sesame seeds
1 cup water, plus 1 to 2 tablespoons
6 tablespoons tamari
1 tablespoon arrowroot or cornstarch

1 Heat the oven to 350°F. Coat the tempeh with olive or sesame oil and sesame seeds. Place the tempeh on a baking sheet and bake in the oven for 45 to 60 minutes, until brown, turning the strips two or three times.

2 For the sauce, heat the oil in a pan and sauté the tomatoes, ginger, and sesame seeds over medium heat for 2 to 3 minutes. Add the 1 cup water and the tamari and simmer for about 10 minutes. Mix the arrowroot with the remaining 1 to 2 tablespoons water and add to the sauce, stirring until it thickens. Serve the sauce with the baked tempeh.

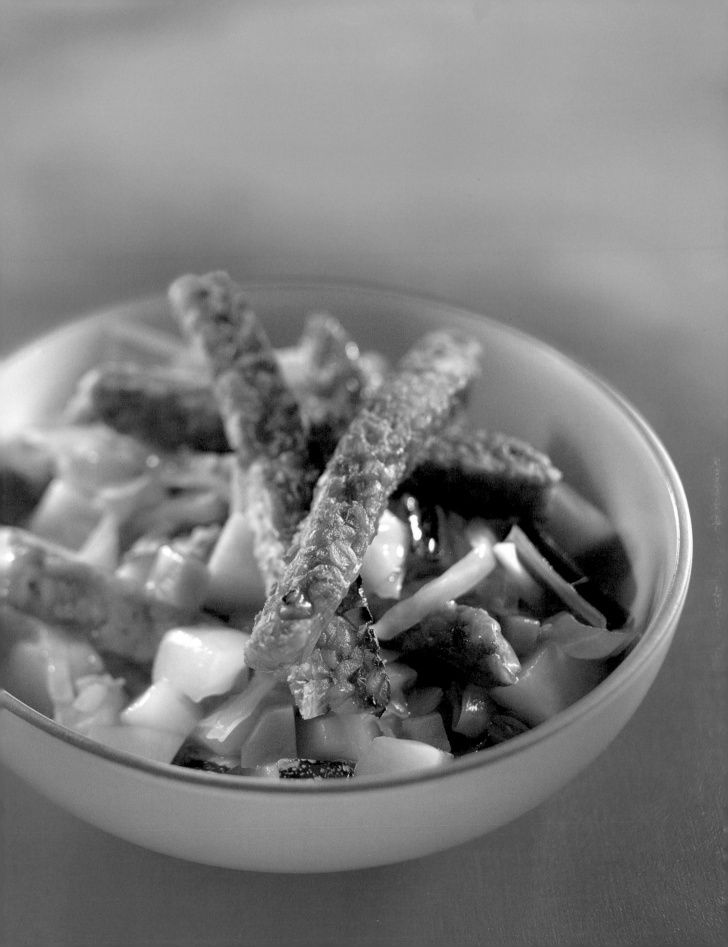

Tofu Also known as bean curd, tofu has become one of the most popular soy foods available. Its versatility and nutritional richness have made it an essential ingredient in vegetarian kitchens. It is extremely high in protein, iron, calcium, and phosphorus, and has very little cholesterol. There are several varieties available, ranging in texture from extra firm to silken. Firm tofu is the most versatile and best for stir-frying and baking. If you are going to make creamier dishes, choose silken tofu, which has a wonderfully smooth texture almost akin to yogurt. Tofu can be used in many recipes as a substitute for dairy products such as cheese and cream, and because of its neutral flavor can be used in both savory and sweet dishes. Buy the freshest available and check the label to make sure genetically modified soybeans have not been used in its manufacture. Keep tofu covered in cold water in the refrigerator. For health reasons, it is best not to eat raw tofu unless you have made it yourself; if using it in uncooked dishes, steam the tofu for a few minutes first.

Crispy Baked Tofu *Serve this tasty bake with brown rice, millet, or any of the grain dishes on pages 47-65.* Serves 4 to 6

1 pound firm tofu	2 to 3 tablespoons tamari
2 to 3 tablespoons butter or margarine	Nutritional yeast flakes for sprinkling

1 Heat the oven to 375°F. Slice the tofu into 8 or 12 pieces.

2 Melt the butter or margarine in a pan, remove it from the heat, and add the tamari.

3 Place the tofu pieces on a baking sheet and brush with the tamari and butter or margarine mixture. Sprinkle with the yeast flakes and bake in the oven for 20 minutes, or until the tofu is lightly roasted and crispy.

• **Baked Marinated Tofu:** For moister tofu with some sauce, combine 2 tablespoons toasted sesame oil or melted butter or margarine, with 2 tablespoons tamari, 2 tablespoons grated gingerroot, and 4 tablespoons water. Pour this mixture over the tofu pieces in a dish and leave to marinate for 1 hour. Place in the oven with the marinade. Cover the dish with a lid or foil and bake as above. Serve with anything.

Tofu-Carrot Mousse *This is a wonderful way to use winter vegetables. Serve with steamed new potatoes and a crisp salad.* Serves 6

2 tablespoons sesame oil	1 to 2 tablespoons tamari
2 to 3 carrots, sliced	9 ounces firm tofu
1 small rutabaga or 1 parsnip, roughly chopped	Toasted sesame seeds or chopped fresh parsley,
½ cup water	to garnish (optional)

1 Heat the oven to 400°F. Heat the sesame oil in a pan and sauté the carrots and rutabaga or parsnip over medium heat for 5 minutes. Add the water and tamari and simmer until the vegetables are tender.

2 Transfer the vegetables to a food processor or blender, add the tofu, and blend until smooth. Spoon the mixture into a 2½-cup baking dish and bake in the oven for about 30 minutes, until just firm. Leave to cool, then garnish with sesame seeds or parsley before serving.

Sweet and Sour Tofu
This is delicious with just a bowl of rice or it can be served as part of a Chinese feast. Serves 4 to 6

1 pound firm tofu
2 tablespoons tamari
Kuzu, arrowroot, or cornstarch for coating
(optional)
4 tablespoons sesame oil
1 green bell pepper, cored, seeded, and chopped
1 stick of celery, cut into 1-inch diagonal slices
1 carrot, sliced diagonally
4 ounces snow peas, sliced diagonally

4 ounces bamboo shoots, cut into wedges
5 ounces water chestnuts, sliced
⅔ cup diced, fresh pineapple
Sauce:
2 tablespoons cornstarch or arrowroot
½ cup water
3 tablespoons honey
4 tablespoons tamari
2 tablespoons lemon juice

1 Wrap the tofu in a clean dish towel. Place a chopping board or heavy book on top and leave for 30 minutes to press out the liquid. Cut the tofu into 1- to 2-inch cubes and sprinkle them with tamari. Coat with kuzu, arrowroot, or cornstarch, if using.

2 Heat 2 tablespoons of the sesame oil in a wok or skillet and fry the tofu until crisp; set aside (preferably keep warm in a low oven).

3 Heat the remaining oil in the wok and stir-fry the green bell pepper, celery, carrot, and snow peas for 5 minutes, until the vegetables are tender but still firm. Stir in the bamboo shoots, water chestnuts, and pineapple and cook for 2 to 3 minutes. Remove the vegetables and keep warm.

4 To make the sauce, dissolve the cornstarch or arrowroot in the water. Combine the remaining sauce ingredients in a separate bowl and add to the wok. When the sauce starts to boil, add the cornstarch or arrowroot mixture and stir for 2 minutes, or until the sauce thickens. Add the fried tofu and vegetables, mix well, and serve at once.

Tofu, Pasta, and Olives
This is tofu in Mediterranean guise, made into a creamy sauce to serve with pasta. Silken tofu is best but the firm variety will do. This quantity of olives gives the sauce a wonderful flavor, but you can reduce the amount or substitute sun-dried tomatoes for some of the olives. Serves 4 to 6

1 pound silken tofu
2 tablespoons olive oil
Scant 1 cup chopped celery
3½ cups chopped kale or spinach
½ teaspoon each of dried basil, oregano,
thyme

1 bay leaf
1 pound dried pasta
4 tablespoons light miso
1½ cups pitted and sliced ripe olives
1½ cups pitted and sliced green olives
Pepper

1 Poach the tofu for 3 minutes in a small pan of simmering water; drain and set aside.

2 Heat the olive oil in a heavy skillet. Add the celery, kale or spinach, dried herbs, and the bay leaf and stir-fry for 3 to 4 minutes, then reduce the heat to low and for cook 6 to 7 minutes longer, or until the celery is soft, stirring occasionally. Discard the bay leaf. Meanwhile, cook the pasta in a large pan of boiling water for 8 to 10 minutes, until *al dente* (tender but firm to the bite).

3 Transfer the vegetable mixture to a food processor or blender, add the tofu and miso, and blend to a smooth and creamy sauce. Stir in the ripe and green olives. Drain the cooked pasta and immediately toss it with the tofu mixture. Season with pepper and serve.

VEGETABLE
VIRYA

"Mother Nature has demonstrated her marvelous skill and power in cultivating these wonderful vegetables for her children in her cosmic garden. How kind and merciful She is; She has compounded and beautifully blended all the essentials of life in various kinds of vegetables to give proper strength, vitality, vigor, and energy to Her children."

Swami Sivananda

Virya is the physical and mental energy that is necessary to prosper in any walk of life. Even for spiritual pursuits, vibrant vitality is a prerequisite. Without it, you cannot penetrate into the hidden depths of the vast ocean of life within and attain the final beatitude. Without good health, you cannot wage war with the turbulent senses and boisterous mind. Inner strength, or virya, is the drive that carries one along the path, bouncing back after failures and maintaining courage through even the most difficult times.

Along with the intake of dietary vitamins that are found so abundantly in vegetables, the yogi, attempting to maintain virya, should also partake of "philosophical vitamins," as expressed by Swami Sivananda:

Vitamin A: adaptability, austerity

Vitamin B: bravery, balance of mind, bhakti (devotion)

Vitamin C: compassion, consideration, charity, courage, cooperation, cleanliness, contemplation, contentment, concentration

Vitamin D: diligence, discipline, detachment

Vitamin E: equanimity, edurance

Vitamin F: faith, forgiveness, friendliness, firmness, fasting, fortitude, fearlessness, forbearance, frankness

Vitamin K: kindness, knowledge

Vitamin P: patience, perseverance, purity, politeness

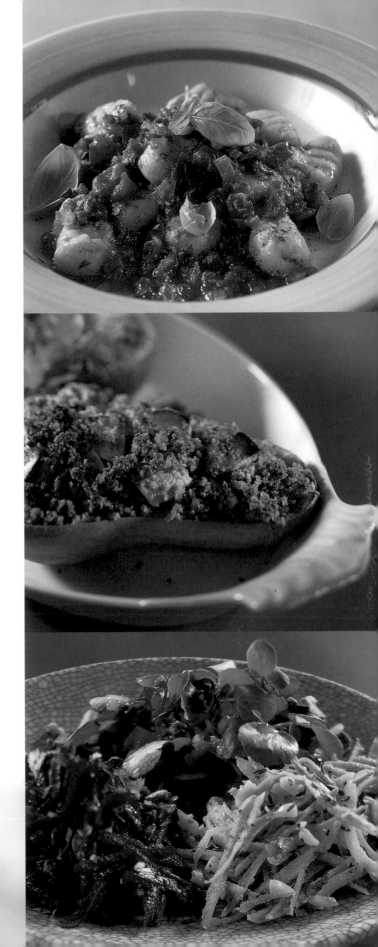

"Vegetables are the most important sources of vitamins in every diet—especially those that can be eaten raw. The humble tomato because of its wealth of the three main types of vitamins (A, B, and C), is considered, along with lettuce, spinach, and cabbage, one of the elect, one of the big four, that head the vegetable kingdom."

Swami Vishnu-devananda

Vegetables are also our main sources of valuable minerals (such as iron and potassium) that act as eliminators, antiseptics, blood purifiers, and producers of electromagnetic energy. They also help to keep an alkaline reserve in the body, which is essential for maintaining the blood's capacity for carrying carbon dioxide to the lungs for elimination. They aid the digestion and assimilation of the proteins in legumes, and supply fiber. Leafy and juicy vegetables help to prevent the blood from becoming too acid by balancing the acid-generating sugars, fats, proteins, and starches.

Steaming is the simplest and healthiest way of cooking vegetables to prevent loss of nutrients, preserving maximum prana, natural flavor, and texture. Wash vegetables in cold water and peel ones like carrots if they are not organic. Vegetables can be cut horizontally or lengthwise; it makes an attractive dish if you vary the types of slices, cubes, and batons. Put about 1 cup water into a wok or steamer and bring to a boil. Place the vegetables in a steamer basket over the water, cover tightly, and steam for 5 to 10 minutes. Do not overcook; steamed vegetables should be crisp and retain their natural color. Vegetables may be steamed individually, or several varieties together. Cook similar types together; for example, root vegetables will need longer than seeded vegetables, and both will need longer than leafy greens.

Stir-frying is another quick, healthy way of cooking vegetables. Allow a good handful of vegetables per person—favorites or seasonal ones. Wash, trim, and cut into bite-size pieces. Vegetables should stay crisp, not become limp and overcooked; cook them in the same order as for steaming.

Vegetables can also be baked; potatoes are the favorite, but other root or strong-flavored vegetables can be baked whole or cut into pieces and baked in foil packages.

Spiced Spring Carrots
This recipe was devised by Jyoti, our Irish teacher at the London center. Carrots are rich in vitamin A, purify the blood, and tone the kidneys. Crushed hazelnuts can be substituted for the almonds. Serves 4

4 carrots, cut into matchsticks
½ cup slivered almonds
4 tablespoons butter or margarine
1 teaspoon ground cumin

2 teaspoons chopped fresh cilantro
1 teaspoon honey
Salt and pepper (optional)

1 Steam the carrot sticks for about 10 minutes, until tender but still crunchy. Meanwhile, set aside a few of the slivered almonds and toast the remainder in a dry, heavy pan over high heat, until golden brown around the edges.

2 Melt the butter or margarine in a pan and cook the cumin over high heat for a few seconds to release the aroma, being careful to not burn it. Take the pan off the heat and add the carrots, browned almonds, and cilantro. Mix well, then stir in the honey. Add a pinch of salt and pepper, if desired. Serve at once, garnished with the reserved almonds.

Exotic Eggplant and Snow Peas *This half-Chinese, half-Indian dish marries the smoothness of eggplant with the crispness of snow peas. This combination of contrasting textures can be seen to symbolize the totality of Nature.* Serves 4

1 eggplant, peeled and cut into ¾-inch
  cubes
Salt (optional)
3 tablespoons oil
1 teaspoon black mustard seeds
1 teaspoon chopped fresh gingerroot
¼ teaspoon ground coriander
¼ teaspoon ground cumin

¼ teaspoon ground turmeric
9 ounces snow peas, sliced diagonally into
  ¾-inch pieces
½ cup water
1 small tomato, chopped
2 teaspoons lemon juice
2 tablespoons tamari

1 If liked, sprinkle the eggplant cubes with salt and leave to drain for 1 hour; rinse and pat dry. (This removes some of the bitterness and cuts down on the oil absorbed.)

2 Heat the oil in a heavy skillet or wok. Add the mustard seeds and ginger and cook over high heat until the mustard seeds "pop." Add the rest of the spices and sauté over medium heat for about 5 minutes. Stir in the eggplant and snow peas, turning them to coat with spices.

3 Add the water, cover, and cook until the vegetables are soft and cooked, at most 8 minutes. Remove from heat and add the chopped tomato, lemon juice, and tamari. Cover the pan again and leave to stand for a few minutes before serving.

Long Beans in Black Bean Sauce *Long beans have more body than common green beans and cooking them in black bean sauce increases the protein value of this vegetable dish. Fresh long beans and salted black beans are available from Chinese food stores. Serve the beans with brown rice for a simple, nourishing meal. For an impressive Chinese meal, serve with Sweet and Sour Tofu (page 81), preceded by Tofu Vegetable Soup Orientale (page 42).* Serves 4 to 6

2 tablespoons oil
1 pound long beans, trimmed and cut into
  2-inch pieces
2 to 3 tablespoons mashed salted black beans
1 tablespoon tamari

1 tablespoon honey
4 tablespoons water, plus 1 tablespoon
1 tablespoon cornstarch or arrowroot
Toasted sesame seeds for sprinkling

1 Heat the oil in a wok or heavy skillet and stir-fry the long beans over high heat for about 2 minutes.

2 Combine the black beans, tamari, honey, and the 4 tablespoons water. Add this mixture to the long beans and cook for 2 minutes.

3 Dissolve the cornstarch or arrowroot in the remaining 1 tablespoon water. Stir it into the beans and cook for 2 minutes. Sprinkle with toasted sesame seeds and serve at once.

• Use green beans instead of long beans.

Gnocchi with Spinach and Basil Sauce

These tender, little Italian dumplings are best when homemade, and make a delightful alternative to pasta dishes. You can use fresh or canned tomatoes. Serves 6

2¼ pounds potatoes, chopped
Salt
1 tablespoon chopped fresh basil
1½ cups whole wheat flour
Water or oil for mixing (optional)
Grated vegetarian cheese, to serve (optional)
Basil leaves, to garnish

Sauce:
1½ tablespoons olive oil
1 to 2 sticks of celery, finely chopped
1¼ pounds plum tomatoes, chopped
1½ tablespoons tomato paste
5 cups finely chopped spinach
2 tablespoons chopped fresh basil or
   3 tablespoons dried basil
Pepper

1 Cook the potatoes in a pan of salted boiling water for 15 minutes, or until tender. Drain and press through a strainer. Stir in the tablespoon of basil and gradually add the flour. Mix to a soft dough, adding a little water or oil if the mixture is too stiff, or more flour if it is too wet.

2 Cool slightly, then knead the dough lightly until smooth. Divide it into quarters and shape each portion into a roll, 16 inches long and 1 inch in diameter. Cut the dough into ¾-inch pieces and press a fork lightly into each one to make a pattern. Place them on a floured surface and leave to dry for 10 to 15 minutes.

3 Meanwhile, make the sauce. Heat the olive oil and sauté the celery until soft. Add the tomatoes, tomato paste, and spinach, and cook, uncovered, over medium heat for 5 to 10 minutes, stirring occasionally. Add the basil and season to taste with salt and pepper; keep warm.

4 Cook the gnocchi, in batches, in boiling water for 2 to 3 minutes, or until they rise to the surface. Keep warm until they are all cooked. Top with the sauce and serve at once. Sprinkle with a little cheese, if desired, and garnish with basil leaves.

Latkes
These potato pancakes, a mainstay of Jewish cuisine, are a wonderful source of energy and are rich in vitamin C and potassium. If you don't want to grate the potatoes and turnips, dice them and then purée in a food processor. Baking the latkes means they are not as crisp as fried ones, but they are less oily. Serve with applesauce and/or sour cream or yogurt. Serves 6

6 potatoes, finely grated
1 large turnip, finely grated
1 teaspoon mustard powder
2 teaspoons baking powder

2½ cups matzo meal, or 2½ cups fresh
   whole wheat bread crumbs, plus a little
   extra if necessary
¼ teaspoon salt

1 Heat the oven to 375°F. Drain the potatoes thoroughly to remove all the excess water. Place them in a bowl and add the turnip, mustard powder, baking powder, matzo meal or bread crumbs, and salt. Mix well, adding more matzo meal or crumbs if necessary to bind.

2 Using your hands, shape the mixture into small patties, about 1¾ inches across. Place them on a baking sheet and bake in the oven for about 20 minutes, until crisp on the bottom. Turn over and bake for 20 minutes longer, until both sides are crisp. They should be crisp on the outside and soft on the inside.

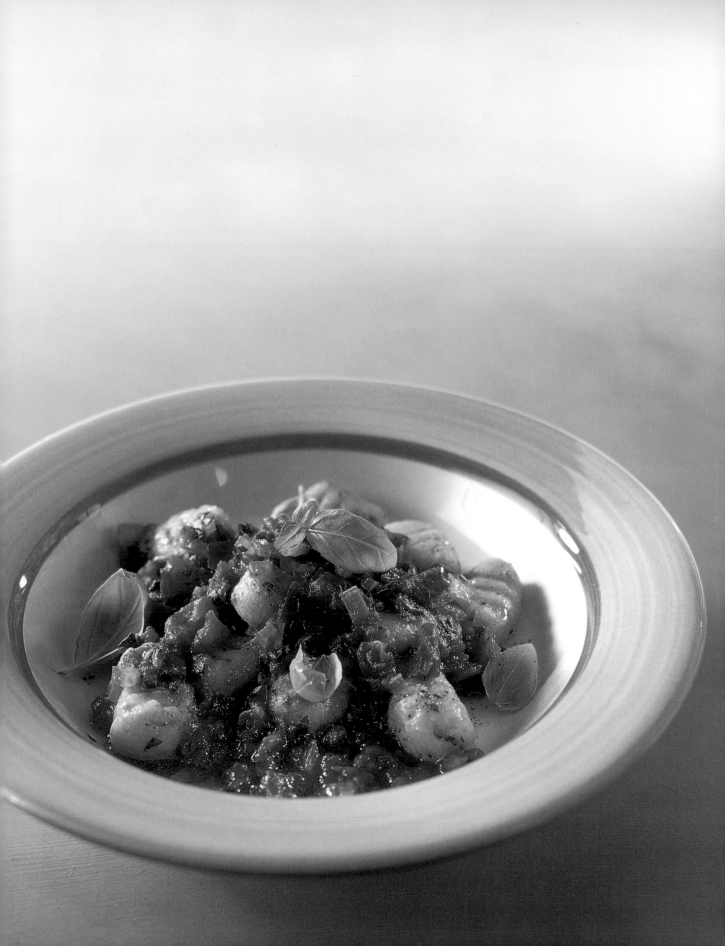

Curried Vegetables

The word "curry" can be used to refer to any dish of vegetables cooked in a spicy sauce. In northern India, the spices are usually cooked in a tomato base. In the south, grated coconut is frequently used instead of tomato. This basic recipe can be adapted to use whatever vegetables you have to hand. It can be served as part of a simple Indian meal with plain rice, Lentil Dal (page 76) and Chapatis (page 53). Serves 4 to 6

2 tablespoons oil	1 cauliflower, separated into small flowerets
1 teaspoon black mustard seeds	2 potatoes, cubed and parboiled
¼ teaspoon turmeric	4 tablespoons water
1 teaspoon curry powder	Lemon juice to taste (optional)
1 tomato, chopped	1 teaspoon salt

1 Heat the oil in a large pan and toast the mustard seeds over high heat until they "pop." Add the turmeric and curry powder and stir well. Reduce the heat, add the chopped tomato, and cook for 3 to 4 minutes, until soft.

2 Add the cauliflower, stirring gently to coat the flowerets with the spices. Stir in the potatoes, water, lemon juice, and salt. Cover and cook for 15 to 20 minutes, until the potatoes and cauliflower are just tender. Add a little more water if necessary to prevent the mixture drying out. Serve hot.

- Omit the cauliflower to use as a traditional stuffing for Masala Dosa (page 28).
- Replace the cauliflower with 10 to 14 ounces vegetables of your choice.

Bavarian Red Cabbage

The deep red of the cabbage with the hint of cloves and cinnamon makes this elegantly simple dish a perennial favorite at the very busy Sivananda Yoga Center in Munich. Serves 4 to 6

1 tablespoon oil, butter, or margarine	2 slivers of cinnamon stick
1 small red cabbage, coarsely shredded	Juice of 1 lemon
1 carrot, grated	½ teaspoon salt
⅔ cup water	Pepper to taste (optional)
6 whole cloves	

Heat the oil, butter, or margarine in a heavy pan and sauté the cabbage and carrot over medium heat for 5 minutes. Add the water and spices. Cover and cook for about 30 minutes, until the cabbage is tender. Season with the lemon juice, salt, and pepper, and serve warm.

- The cabbage and spices can be baked in a 350°F oven instead of on the stovetop, if preferred.

Indian-Style Cabbage
This delicately spiced dish goes well with Lentil Dal (page 76) and plain rice or Chapatis (see page 53). For a more elegant North Indian meal, serve it with Rice Pilau (page 47) and Curried Vegetables (see opposite), using zucchini instead of cauliflower. Serves 4 to 6

1 potato, diced
2 tablespoons oil or ghee (or half and half)
1 tablespoon mustard seeds
1½ teaspoons cumin seeds
1 teaspoon ground coriander

½ teaspoon turmeric
Dash of cayenne pepper
1 cabbage, finely chopped
1 teaspoon salt

1 Steam the diced potato for 5 to 10 minutes to part-cook; set aside. Heat the oil in a heavy skillet. Add the mustard seeds and cook over high heat until they "pop." Add the other spices and sauté over medium heat for 1 to 2 minutes.

2 Add the cabbage, stir well, and cook until the cabbage is soft. Add the part-cooked potatoes and salt and cook for about 5 minutes, until the potatoes are cooked; the dish should be fairly dry. Serve at once.

Ratatouille
All the vegetables can be sautéed together if you are in a hurry, but the flavor is best if you roast the eggplant and zucchini first to bring out their very distinctive flavors. The grated carrot is added to balance the acidity of the tomatoes. Serve the ratatouille over pasta or rice and sprinkle with grated vegetarian cheese, if desired. For a complete meal, serve with a green salad as well.
Serves 4 to 6

1 eggplant, cut into large chunks
2 to 3 zucchini, cut into large chunks
Extra-virgin olive oil
Salt and pepper
2 sticks of celery, finely chopped
1 red bell pepper, cored, seeded, and
   cut into strips

1 carrot, grated
3 large juicy tomatoes, chopped
1 tablespoon tomato paste
2 tablespoons chopped fresh basil or
   1 tablespoon dried oregano or basil

1 Heat the oven to 400°F. Place the eggplant and zucchini in a baking dish greased with olive oil. Brush with more olive oil, sprinkle with salt and pepper, and bake in the oven for 20 to 30 minutes, until the vegetables are tender.

2 Meanwhile, heat 1 tablespoon of olive oil in a pan and sauté the celery over medium heat for 2 to 3 minutes. Add the red bell pepper and cook until soft. Add the grated carrot, tomatoes, tomato paste, and herbs and cook for 5 minutes.

3 Add the tomato mixture to the baked vegetables. Taste and adjust the seasoning, if necessary, before serving.

Baked Butternut Squash
This is a cool-weather favorite at the Sivananda Yoga Ranch in upstate New York. Butternut squash has a glorious color reminiscent of the glowing fall foliage, and its creamy, sweet flavor enlivens any meal on a cold evening. Rich in vitamin A, squash is also known to soothe acidic stomachs and help counteract the effects of ill-considered foods. Serves 4 to 6

1 butternut squash or 2 acorn squash
4 tablespoons butter or margarine, melted
2 cups fresh whole wheat bread crumbs
¼ teaspoon freshly grated nutmeg

½ teaspoon ground cinnamon
2 large eating apples, peeled and cut into chunks

1 Heat the oven to 350°F. Cut the squash in half and remove the seeds and stringy bits.

2 Mix the melted butter or margarine with the bread crumbs, spices, and apples and spoon this mixture into the squash halves. Place them in a roasting pan, cover with foil, and bake for about 45 minutes. Remove the foil and bake 10 minutes longer to brown the tops. Serve hot.

Creamy Baked Fennel
Fennel is a diuretic and helps to clear the lungs. Here, its delicate licorice flavor is complemented by cheese and caraway seeds. Serves 4

2 bulbs of fennel
2 tablespoons lemon juice
2 teaspoons caraway seeds
2 tablespoons butter or margarine
2 cups fresh bread crumbs

¾ cup plus 2 tablespoons drained ricotta cheese
⅔ cup milk or soy milk
1 teaspoon salt
1 tablespoon chopped fresh parsley

1 Heat the oven to 400°F. Slice the fennel thinly, reserving the feathery fronds for garnishing. Place the slices in a pan and pour the lemon juice over them. Cover and steam over medium heat for 5 to 10 minutes, until the fennel begins to soften.

2 Meanwhile, toast the caraway seeds in a dry skillet over high heat for a few seconds and then crush them slightly. Melt the butter or margarine in a pan and fry the bread crumbs over medium heat until lightly brown.

3 Transfer the fennel to a 6¼-cup baking dish. Beat together the ricotta cheese, milk, caraway seeds, and salt, then pour the mixture over the fennel. Sprinkle the bread crumbs on top and then the chopped parsley. Cover with foil and bake for 25 to 30 minutes, until the fennel is tender. Serve hot.

• For a vegan version of this dish, substitute silken tofu for the ricotta cheese.

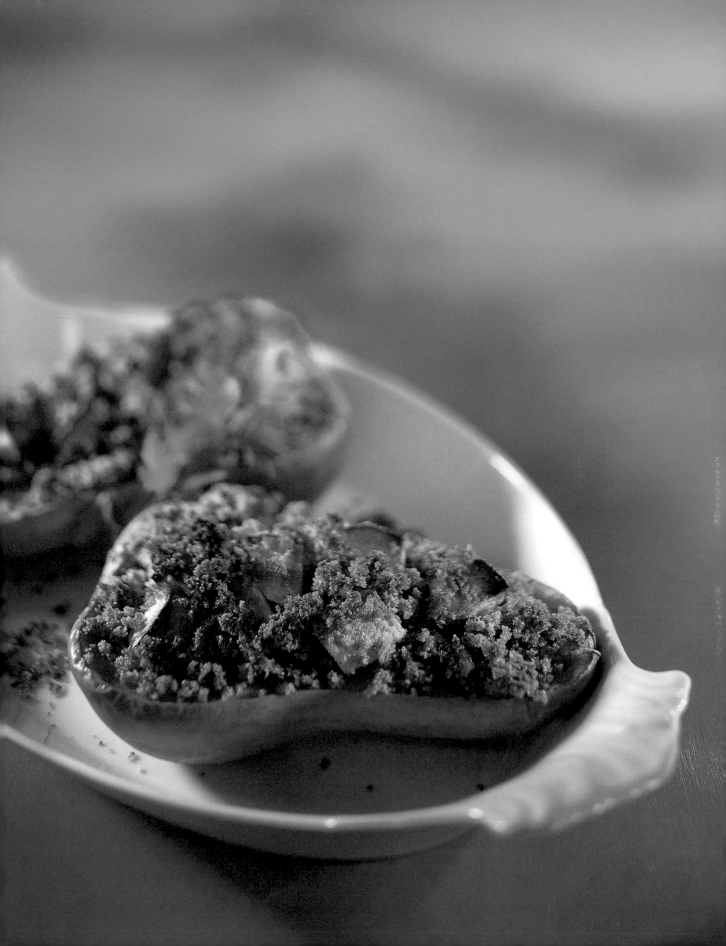

Gobi Masala *Special thanks to Shakti Warwick; her innovative recipe is a feast for the eyes as well as the palate. A whole cauliflower is cooked Indian style to make a deliciously tangy dish. For a milder flavor, reduce the spices or add more yogurt. Serve with just rice or as part of a larger meal.* Serves 4

1 cauliflower
1 fresh green chili, seeded and finely chopped
½ teaspoon cayenne pepper
¾ teaspoon salt
1 teaspoon grated fresh gingerroot
½ teaspoon garam masala,
　plus ½ teaspoon for sprinkling
1 teaspoon lemon juice
Chopped cilantro leaves or parsley, to garnish
Masala paste:
½ cup melted ghee or oil
2 sticks of celery, finely sliced
1 very small white turnip, finely grated
1 tablespoon grated fresh gingerroot

2 tablespoons unsweetened dried
　coconut
½ cup almonds, finely ground
2 tablespoons ground coriander
½ teaspoon cumin seeds
6 whole cloves
8 peppercorns
4 green cardamoms, seeded and husk discarded
Pinch of freshly grated nutmeg
¾-inch piece of cinnamon stick
¾ teaspoon salt
4 tablespoons plain yogurt
1 small tomato, seeded and finely chopped

1 Heat the oven to 350°F. Wash and dry the cauliflower and remove the outer leaves.

2 Using a spice grinder or mortar and pestle, grind the chili, cayenne pepper, ¾ teaspoon salt, 1 teaspoon grated ginger, and ½ teaspoon garam masala with the lemon juice to make a paste. Force the paste between the cauliflower flowerets without breaking them off. Place the cauliflower in a steamer basket and steam for 8 to 10 minutes, until about three-quarters cooked.

3 Meanwhile, make the masala paste. Reserve 2 tablespoons of the ghee or oil. Heat the rest in a skillet and sauté the celery and turnip. Grind the grated ginger, coconut, almonds, spices, and salt together. Stir this mixture into the vegetables. Cook for a moment or two, then slowly add the yogurt, stirring to prevent it from separating. Stir in the chopped tomato.

4 Place the steamed cauliflower in a baking dish. Cover the top with half the masala paste, using your hands to push the paste down into the crevices of the vegetable. Drizzle the reserved ghee or oil over. Bake the cauliflower in the oven for 15 minutes, or until the masala is brown and evenly cooked.

5 Pour the remaining masala paste around the cauliflower and bake for 5 minutes longer. To serve, sprinkle the cauliflower with the remaining garam masala and garnish with the chopped cilantro or parsley.

Vegetable Ragout

A simple and satisfying winter vegetable dish, retaining all the goodness of the vegetables in the liquid. The addition of dill enhances the flavor of the vegetables. Serve over brown rice with a fresh green salad. Serves 4

3 sticks of celery	1 tablespoon oil, butter, or margarine
2 or 3 potatoes	6 tomatoes, cut into wedges
2 or 3 carrots	Salt and pepper to taste
2 or 3 zucchini	3 tablespoons chopped fresh dill

1 Heat the oven to 350°F. Chop all the vegetables into large chunks.

2 Heat the oil or butter or margarine in a pan and sauté the celery over medium heat for about 5 minutes, until it has softened slightly.

3 Place all the chopped vegetables and the tomato wedges in a shallow baking dish, season with salt and pepper, and sprinkle with 2 tablespoons of the dill. Pour in enough water to cover the bottom of the dish.

4 Bake in the oven for about 1 hour, until tender, stirring from time to time. Add a little more water if it starts to dry out and cover with a lid or foil, if necessary. Serve with the remaining dill sprinkled over the top.

Walnut and Potato Bake

Make sure you buy nuts from a food store with a fast turnover so they are not stale. Look for ones that are not coated with additives. Serve this baked dish with steamed vegetables and a green salad for a simple, yet elegant meal. Serves 4 to 6

3 cups scrubbed but not peeled and roughly chopped potatoes	¼ cup milk or soy milk
1 tablespoon butter or oil	½ cup chopped walnuts
2 cups grated vegetarian cheese, or ½ ounce nutritional yeast flakes	Tamari to taste
	¼ teaspoon paprika
	Chopped fresh parsley, to garnish

1 Heat the oven to 350°F. Steam the potatoes until tender, then mash them and add the butter or oil and grated cheese or yeast flakes; mix well.

2 Stir in the milk or soy milk, chopped walnuts, and tamari to taste. Mix well and transfer to a greased baking dish. Sprinkle with the paprika and bake in the oven for 20 minutes. Garnish with chopped parsley and serve at once.

Baked Stuffed Tomatoes
Rich in vitamins and minerals, tomatoes are a great accompaniment to any meal. If possible, use vine-ripened tomatoes because their flavor is so good. Serve these stuffed tomatoes with a simple green salad or lightly steamed green vegetables for a light lunch or supper, or with Mediterranean Salad (page 98) for a more substantial meal. Serves 4 to 6

6 to 8 tomatoes
4 tablespoons oil
1 turnip, grated
½ cup chopped walnuts
1 tablespoon chopped fresh dill or 1 teaspoon dried dillweed

1 tablespoon chopped fresh parsley
¾ cup fresh whole wheat bread crumbs, or ¼ cup cooked brown rice or other grain
¼ teaspoon pepper
1 teaspoon tamari

1 Heat the oven to 350°F. Cut a slice off each tomato to make a lid and reserve. Scoop out the pulp using a teaspoon; set aside.

2 Heat half the oil in a pan and cook the turnip until brown. Add the tomato pulp and sauté for 1 to 2 minutes. Add the chopped walnuts, dill, parsley, bread crumbs or rice, and pepper and sauté for 3 minutes. Stir in the tamari. Spoon the stuffing into the tomatoes. Cover with the reserved "lids" and sprinkle with the remaining oil.

3 Place the filled tomatoes in a shallow baking dish and add enough water to cover the bottom of the dish. Bake in the oven for 30 to 40 minutes, then serve hot.

Eggplant Pizzas
Serve hot from the oven as a snack or add a grain dish and salad for a full meal. Serves 4 to 6

1 large eggplant
4 teaspoons sesame seeds
4 teaspoons dried oregano
4 teaspoons dried basil
Salt to taste

⅔ cup olive oil
2 or 3 large tomatoes, sliced
1 cup grated vegetarian cheese and/or vegetarian mozzarella cheese

1 Heat the oven to 350°F. Slice the eggplant into ½-inch slices. Combine the sesame seeds, dried herbs, and salt on a plate. Brush the eggplant slices with oil and then dredge in the sesame seed mixture until coated.

2 Place each slice on a greased baking sheet and top with a slice of tomato and some grated cheese. Bake in the oven for about 30 minutes, or until the eggplant is tender. Serve hot.

• For a vegan version of this dish, substitute 7 ounces firm tofu for the cheese. Slice the tofu and marinate it in a mixture of 3 tablespoons tamari, 3 tablespoons water, and 1 tablespoon grated gingerroot before adding to the pizzas.
• Sliced olives and/or other toppings may be added before or after baking.

Shepherd's Pie
This is a delicious meal, combining high-protein lentils with carbohydrate-rich potato topping. Lentils are also rich in iron and one of the easiest legumes to prepare and digest. This pie can be served plain with a simple green salad. Serves 4 to 6

1½ cups green or brown lentils
3 cups hot water
2 tablespoons butter or margarine
1 green bell pepper, cored, seeded, and chopped
1 red bell pepper, cored, seeded, and chopped
2 carrots, chopped
2 sticks of celery, chopped
1 teaspoon Italian seasoning
¼ teaspoon ground mace or nutmeg (optional)
¼ teaspoon cayenne pepper

½ teaspoon salt, or 1 teaspoon tamari
2 tomatoes, sliced
Chopped fresh parsley
Potato topping:
1½ pounds potatoes, cooked
¾ cup grated vegetarian cheese (optional)
4 tablespoons butter or margarine
2 tablespoons milk or soy milk
Salt and pepper
Paprika for sprinkling (optional)

1 Put the lentils in a pan with the hot water. Bring to a boil, half cover, and simmer for 30 to 40 minutes, until the water has been absorbed and the lentils are soft.

2 Heat the oven to 375°F. Melt the butter or margarine in a skillet and sauté the peppers, carrots, and celery over medium heat until soft. Mash the cooked lentil, and add to the vegetables. Add the herbs, spices, and salt or tamari; mix well. Spoon the mixture into a deep 2-quart baking dish, arrange the sliced tomatoes on top, and sprinkle with the parsley.

3 To make the topping, mash the cooked potatoes with the cheese, butter, and milk or soy milk. Season with salt and pepper. Spoon the potato over the lentil mixture and sprinkle with paprika, if desired. Bake in the oven for about 30 minutes, until the top is golden brown. Serve hot.

• Adzuki beans or green or yellow split peas may be used instead of all, or some of, the lentils.
• Make the topping with a mixture of rutabaga, potatoes, and parsnip.
• Sprinkle sunflower seeds over the potato, instead of paprika.

Salads
Raw vegetables should be a major component of any healthy diet. Use whatever vegetables are in season. Try not to combine too many different food groups and avoid eating raw vegetables and fruits in the same meal. Leafy green vegetables are a great blessing to humanity; they imbibe the maximum qualities of sunlight and air. They are the lungs and liver of the plants, Nature's storehouse of vitamins and minerals. Green has great power as a healing color. Eaten fresh and in season, salads add variety, texture and taste to any meal. Serves 4 to 6

1 romaine lettuce, torn into bite-size pieces
1 bunch of watercress, coarsely chopped

3 cups spinach or Belgian endive, torn into bite-size pieces
Salad dressing of your choice (pages 118-120)

Combine the lettuce, watercress, and spinach or endive in a salad bowl. Just before serving, pour the dressing over and toss the salad to coat the leaves in dressing.

• Add any combination of the following: chopped fresh herbs; leafy salad vegetables and/or sprouts; lightly steamed or raw vegetables, such as green beans, fava beans or peas, chopped celery or fennel.

Tricolor Salad
This healthy salad platter makes a splendid centerpiece for a festive occasion. The colors are stunning. Serves 4 to 6

Red—Beet salad:
4 raw beets, grated
Generous 1 cup sunflower seeds, toasted
1 tablespoon chopped fresh thyme or tarragon
1 cup Eggless Mayonnaise (page 120)
Green—Watercress salad:
1 cup walnut pieces
1 bunch of watercress, trimmed
1 green bell pepper, cored, seeded, and sliced
Juice of 1 grapefruit
½ cup olive oil
Salt and pepper to taste

Orange—Carrot salad, Indian style:
2 carrots, shredded
1 teaspoon salt (optional)
1 tablespoon raw unsalted peanuts
1 tablespoon oil
½ teaspoon cumin seeds
½ teaspoon black mustard seeds
1 teaspoon sesame seeds
Pinch of ground coriander
¼ teaspoon cayenne pepper
1 teaspoon lemon or lime juice
2 tablespoons chopped fresh cilantro

1 To make the beet salad, combine all the ingredients.

2 To make the watercress salad, heat a heavy skillet and toast the walnuts over high heat until brown; leave to cool. Mix with the watercress and green bell pepper. In a separate bowl, combine the grapefruit juice, olive oil, salt, and pepper and pour over the watercress mixture.

3 To make the carrot salad, place the carrots in a bowl and stir in the salt. Toast the peanuts in the skillet, stirring constantly, until they turn a darker color and give off a rich aroma. Leave the peanuts to cool and grind them coarsely or crush with a mortar and pestle. Heat the oil in a small pan and toast all the seeds until they "pop." Add the ground coriander and cayenne pepper to the seeds and cook for 1 minute, stirring constantly. Stir the mixture into the carrots, along with the peanuts, lemon or lime juice, and chopped cilantro.

4 Arrange each salad attractively on a large serving platter, keeping them separate.

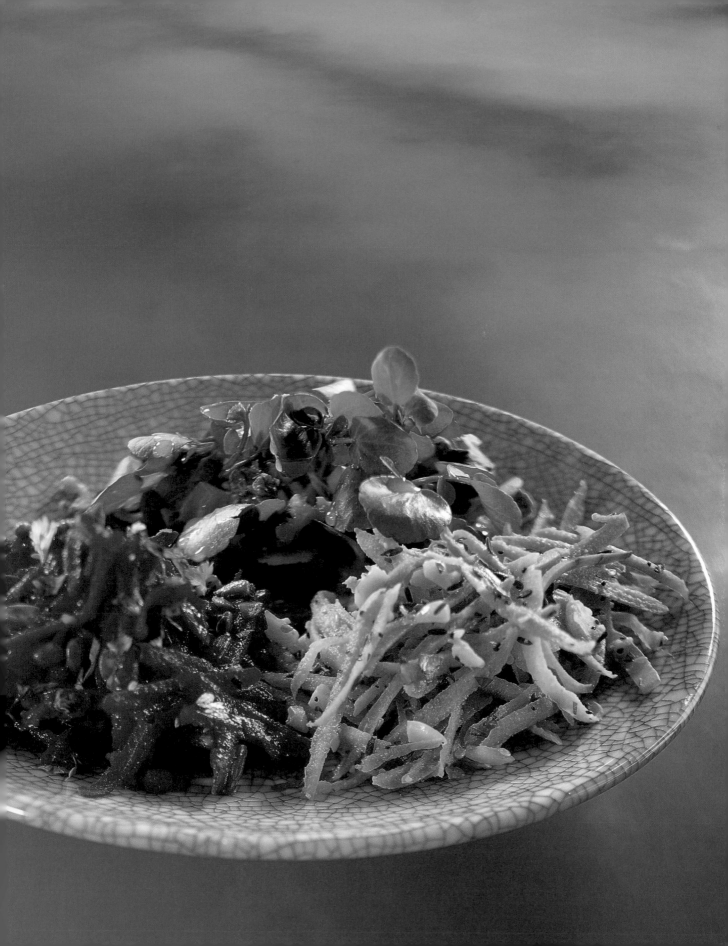

Mediterranean Salad
Feta cheese and olives add piquancy to this attractive salad, and celery gives it a crunchy texture. These quantities will serve four people as a light main course or up to 10 people as a side salad. Serves 4

1 to 2 tablespoons lemon juice
1 to 2 tablespoons olive oil
½ teaspoon dried oregano
½ tablespoon fennel seeds, crushed
A few sprigs of fresh cilantro, finely chopped
¼ teaspoon salt
Pepper to taste
20 ripe olives, pitted
4 ounces romaine lettuce and/or spinach, torn into small pieces

10 ounces green beans, lightly steamed
2 tomatoes, cut into eight wedges, or 10 cherry tomatoes
1 cucumber, cut into chunks
3 carrots, cut into thin sticks about 2 inches long
3 sticks of celery, coarsely chopped
1 cup cubed or crumbled feta cheese, or generous 1 cup sunflower seeds
Few sprigs of fresh parsley, to garnish

1 Combine the lemon juice, olive oil, oregano, fennel seeds, cilantro, salt, and pepper in a small bowl; set aside to let the flavors blend while assembling the rest of the salad.

2 Mix the olives and vegetables together in a large salad bowl. Add the feta cheese or sunflower seeds and the dressing; mix well. Serve garnished with sprigs of parsley.

Coleslaw
Ideal for when you are eating al fresco, this salad is best made a few hours in advance and kept in the refrigerator to let the vegetables absorb the dressing. The red cabbage is not essential, but it adds a lovely color. Serves 6 to 8

1 white cabbage
½ red cabbage (optional)
2 carrots
1 green or red bell pepper (or ½ of each)
1 cup Eggless Mayonnaise (page 120)

1 tablespoon lemon juice
2 tablespoons caraway seeds, toasted (optional)
1 teaspoon salt
Toasted sunflower seeds, to garnish

Shred the white and red cabbages, carrots, and pepper, using a food processor or hand grater. Add the mayonnaise, lemon juice, and caraway seeds, if using. Season to taste with salt. Transfer to a salad bowl. When ready to serve, sprinkle the toasted sunflower seeds over the top.

• **Fennel Coleslaw:** Replace half the shredded cabbage with shredded fennel and add 1 teaspoon toasted fennel seeds. Use 1 tablespoon walnut oil in the dressing, if you have some. Garnish with fennel fronds and chopped walnuts.

Potato Salad
An essential on a traditional summer picnic, potato salad is easy to prepare. Add a few capers or chopped fresh dill for extra zest. Serves 4 to 6

4 to 6 potatoes, scrubbed and cubed
1 teaspoon salt
1 green or red bell pepper, cored, seeded, and diced (optional)

1 stick of celery, chopped (optional)
½ teaspoon paprika
1 cup Eggless Mayonnaise (page 120)

Cook the potatoes in boiling salted water until tender; do not overcook. Drain and leave to cool. When cool, add the other ingredients and toss gently, taking care not to break up the potatoes too much. Serve chilled.

• **German Hot Potato Salad:** Cook 2¼ pounds new potatoes until tender and then slice. While still hot, cover with a little olive oil and lemon juice. Add 1 tablespoon each of chopped fresh mint, parsley, and/or dill. Season with salt and pepper. Serve hot.

Sprouts For year-round, fresh, prana-drenched vegetables, nothing beats sprouts. They can be grown anywhere—one of our staff grew a continuous supply in his backpack as he traveled around India for 2 months. However, sprouting is easier on a non-moving windowsill. As sprouts germinate, the fat and starch content decrease, while protein, chlorophyll, and vitamin C increase. It takes 3 to 7 days for most sprouts to reach optimum nutritional value.

You can buy sprouting trays at most health-food stores, but the easiest method is to use a large glass jar. Soak the beans, grains, or seeds in water overnight. In the morning, secure a piece of cheesecloth over the opening, drain the water, and leave the jar draining at a 45° angle. Rinse the sprouts two or three times a day, draining through the cheesecloth. Mung and Puy lentils take 2 to 3 days and do not need sun at all. Alfalfa takes 5 to 7 days—after 3 days, put the jar in a sunny place so the maximum chlorophyll is formed in the sprouts. Gelatinous seeds, such as cress and flax, do not grow well in a jar. Soak them overnight, then place on two or three layers of paper towels on a plate and water two or three times daily. Grains also seem to prefer this method, taking 4 to 5 days to sprout. They taste very sweet as most of the starch is converted to natural sugars during sprouting. They can be used raw or steamed with a little water for 1 to 2 minutes.

Sprouts Salad
A few sprouts will add a crunchy texture to any vegetable salad, but they also make an excellent main ingredient for a salad. The ingredients given here are per person—simply multiply the ingredients by the number of diners. Any dressing of your choice (pages 118-120) can be drizzled over the sprouts. Recipe per person

1 to 2 ounces sprouts
1 to 2 ounces raw vegetable(s), chopped or shredded

1 carrot, grated
½ tomato, sliced (optional)

Place the sprouts in a large bowl and stir in the chopped or shredded vegetables, grated carrot, and tomato slices, if using. Serve with a little dressing drizzled over the top.

SATTVIC
SWEETS

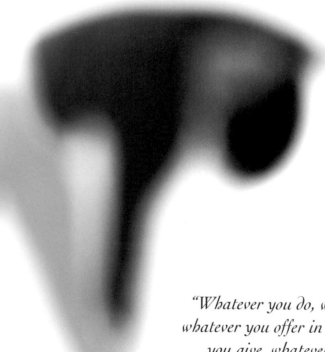

"Whatever you do, whatever you eat,
whatever you offer in sacrifice, whatever
you give, whatever you practice,
do it as an offering to Me."

Bhagavad Gita, IX. 27

At the end of any satsang, prasad (blessed food) is distributed. No spiritual event is considered to be complete unless physical food is offered and consumed. The concept of prasad is like the taking of communion in a church. Food, the carrier of love, is first offered to God to be blessed by God and, after this symbolic gesture, is consumed by the participants.

Prasad is food that has been prepared with love by a person who is practicing Karma Yoga (selfless service). It is prepared fresh (no more than 2 or 3 hours before serving), using the best ingredients. It is kept covered and is NEVER tasted before offering. Even a person who is fasting should accept a small piece, as God's Grace should not be refused.

Prasad may be any type of dish, but it is usually sweet, symbolizing the sweetness of God's Grace. Among our Sattvic Sweets, some are traditional prasads and others are more conventional desserts. In a greater sense, any food that is cooked and offered with love may also be seen as prasad.

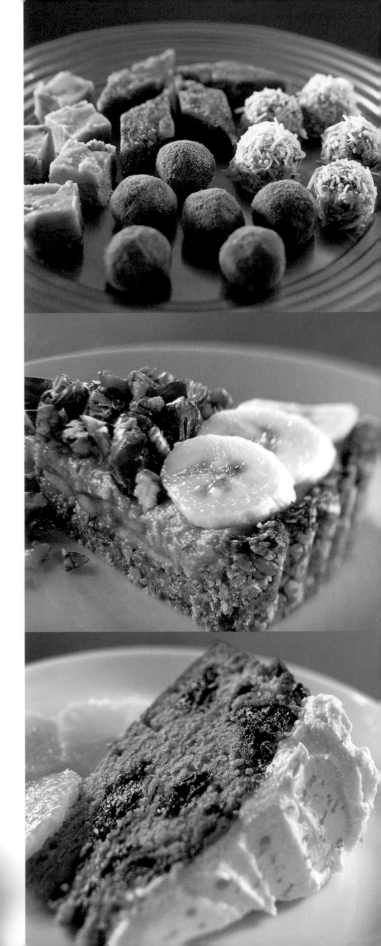

Raisin-Nut Balls
It is the custom at our Christmas parties for everyone to make something. This no-cook recipe is a favorite with the people who think they can't cook, yet want to contribute something. Makes 12

½ cup raisins
⅓ cup unsalted nuts, such as almonds or hazelnuts

4 tablespoons butter, melted
⅓ cup unpacked unsweetened dried coconut

1 Chop the raisins in a food processor or blender to a medium fine mixture and transfer to a bowl. Add the nuts to the food processor or blender and chop to a fairly fine mixture. Mix the nuts into the raisins in the bowl. Stir in the melted butter and mix well.

2 Form the mixture into small balls. Spread the coconut out on a plate and roll the balls in the coconut until coated. They can be eaten straightaway or chilled before serving.

• Substitute peanut butter or tahini for the melted butter.
• Substitute 2 tablespoons honey for the raisins and double the amount of coconut.
• Add ½ teaspoon grated lemon zest.
• Toast the coconut before rolling the balls in it.
• Roll the balls in carob powder instead of coconut.

Chocolate Truffles
These truffles, created by Prema, one of our affiliated teachers in London, are irresistible. They are outrageously sweet, the perfect prasad. Makes 20 large or 40 small

2¼ cups confectioners' sugar
½ cup chopped nuts
2 tablespoons unsweetened cocoa powder
4 tablespoons margarine

1 teaspoon vanilla extract
1 to 2 tablespoons soy milk
Hot chocolate mix for coating

1 Combine the confectioners' sugar, chopped nuts, cocoa powder, margarine, and vanilla extract in a bowl. Slowly add the soy milk; the mixture should be sticky, but not runny.

2 Chill until firm, then form the mixture into small balls. Coat with the hot chocolate mix and keep in the refrigerator or a cool place until ready to serve.

• Ground almonds and almond extract may be substituted for the chopped nuts and vanilla extract.
• Substitute ½ cup unpacked unsweetened dried coconut for the chopped nuts.
• Replace the vanilla extract with 1 teaspoon orange juice and 1 teaspoon finely grated orange zest.

Clockwise from top: Hindustani Halva, Raisin Nut Balls, Chocolate Truffles, Burfi

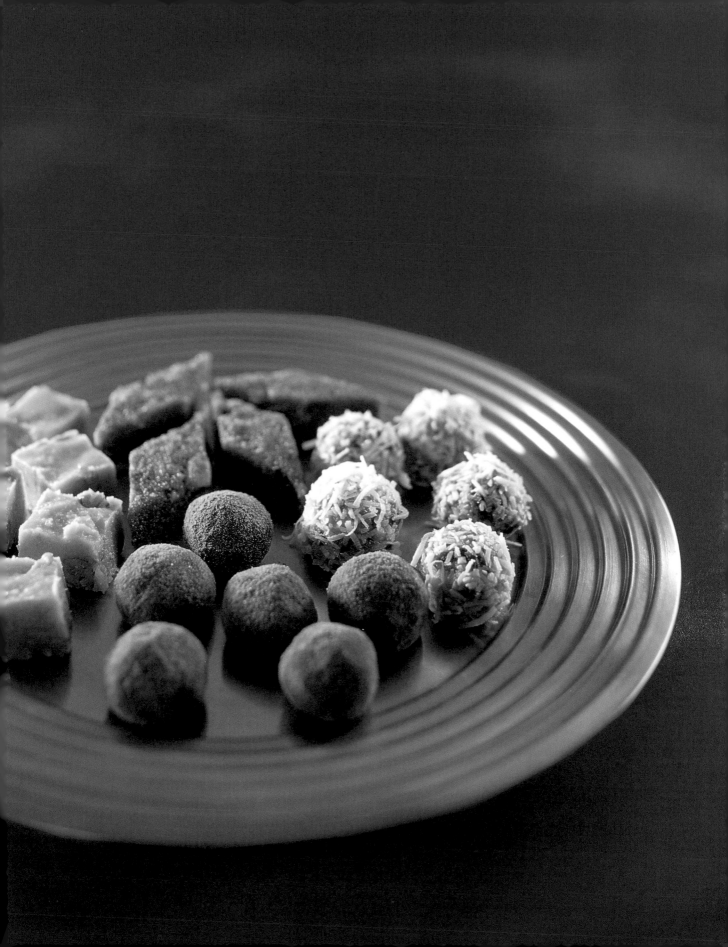

Hindustani Halva

Semolina is one of the most common prasad ingredients, linked with religious ceremonies such as the nine-night holiday of "Navaratri" in October. Halva is also often served warm as a breakfast treat. Serves 16 to 20

1¾ cups semolina
4 tablespoons unsalted butter
⅓ cup cashew nuts (optional)
1 cup packed brown sugar

1 cup water
1 teaspoon ground cardamom
⅓ cup raisins (optional)

1 Toast the semolina in a hot, dry skillet over high heat for 5 minutes, stirring constantly until it turns light brown and gives off a nutty aroma. Stir in the butter and set aside. If using cashews, toast them in a hot, dry pan until lightly brown; set aside.

2 Put the sugar and water in a pan and bring to a boil. Reduce the heat and stir in the semolina, ground cardamom, raisins, and cashews, if using. Continue to cook, stirring continuously, until the mixture thickens.

3 Remove from the heat and spread the mixture evenly on a serving plate. Leave to cool, then score into diamond shapes to make serving easier. Serve with a spoon.

Burfi

This version of the favorite Indian dessert was developed at the Sivananda Yoga Centre in Toronto. Batches were made weekly and delivered to fashionable restaurants and cafés in the city. It's a very rich dessert served in small squares. Use the whole milk powder available from Indian stores and health-food stores, rather than the instant, freeze-dried kind found in supermarkets. Serves 16 to 20

1 cup plus 2 tablespoons butter, at room
   temperature
1¾ cups honey
1 cup walnut pieces

½ teaspoon ground cardamom
4 cups whole milk powder
A little water or milk, if necessary

1 Break up the butter and melt it in a skillet over low heat, but do not allow it to cook because it will separate. Remove from the heat, add the honey, and stir.

2 Using a wooden spoon, stir in the nuts, cardamom, and milk powder, adding a little water or milk if necessary to dissolve all the powdered milk. The consistency should be firm enough for the spoon to stand up straight in the mixture when you let it go.

3 Spread the mixture in a serving dish and chill until set. Remove from the refrigerator 30 minutes before serving to let it come to room temperature. Serve cut into small squares, about 2 inches square.

• Substitute other nuts, such as almonds or pistachios, for the walnuts.
• Add 1 to 2 saffron strands with the honey.

Sunflower-Raisin Cream Pudding *Very sattvic, simple and quick to make, this is a delight for busy people. The pudding can be served on its own or with Raisin Sauce or Raspberry Sauce (pages 114 and 115).* Serves 4

1¾ cups sunflower seeds
⅔ cup raisins

1¼ cups water

1 Put the sunflower seeds, raisins, and water in a pan and cook the mixture over medium heat for 15 to 20 minutes.

2 Transfer the mixture to a food processor or blender and blend to a coarse or a smooth purée. Serve warm or cold.

Banana-Berry Delight *A sumptuous pudding that is easy to make. Bananas are believed to increase humility and strawberries to enhance kindness. Chocolate, high in magnesium, is said to help relax the muscles. You can substitute shredded sweetened coconut for the chocolate to make this a super healthy "delight."* Serves 4 to 6

3 or 4 ripe bananas
1 tablespoon lemon juice
½ cup oil
4 ounces semisweet chocolate, grated

10 ounces firm tofu, steamed
2 tablespoons honey
1¾ cups sliced ripe strawberries or
 other berries

1 Put all the ingredients, except the berries, in a food processor or blender, adding them one at a time and blending before each addition until the mixture is smooth and creamy. Transfer the mixture to a serving dish and stir in the sliced berries. Chill before serving.

Apple Kanten *One of macrobiotic chef Nigel Walker's very sattvic recipes. This traditional macrobiotic dessert is a thick, jellylike custard. It is usually served alone, but is lovely served with Fragrant Fruit Salad (page 145).* Serves 4 to 6

6⅔ cups apple juice
3 tablespoons barley malt or rice syrup
2 teaspoons vanilla extract
3 tablespoons finely grated lemon zest

6 tablespoons agar-agar flakes
Pinch of sea salt
1¼ cups peeled and chopped eating apple

1 Place all the ingredients, except the apple, in a pan and bring to a boil, stirring. Reduce the heat and simmer for 10 to 15 minutes, stirring occasionally.

2 Pour the liquid into a serving bowl and leave to cool for about 20 minutes. Stir in the chopped apple. Leave to cool, stirring once or twice to make sure the lemon zest is distributed evenly throughout. Chill for 1 to 2 hours until softly set.

• Substitute orange juice for apple juice, orange zest for lemon, and 1 teaspoon ginger juice (from fresh gingerroot) and ¼ teaspoon ground cinnamon for the vanilla extract.
• To make a thicker pudding, add 2 tablespoons arrowroot to a little of the cold apple juice and stir it into the pan while the mixture is being heating.

Chocolate & Chick-Pea Mousse

Don't be put off by the unusual ingredients in this recipe. It is an incredibly delicious and lowfat mousse. Serve plain or decorated with fruit and/or ice cream. Serves 8

¾ cup plus 2 tablespoons plain yogurt
1 teaspoon baking soda
2 cups cooked chick-peas, drained (about
  1 cup uncooked)

6 tablespoons orange juice
1⅓ cups unpacked light brown sugar
3 tablespoons unsweetened cocoa powder
1 teaspoon baking powder

1 Heat the oven to 350°F. Grease an 8-inch round cake pan. Mix the yogurt and baking soda together and leave to fizz for 10 minutes.

2 Put the chick-peas and orange juice in a food processor or blender (a food processor is best) and blend until smooth. Add the sugar, cocoa, and baking powder and blend until smooth. Gently fold the yogurt mixture into the chick-pea mixture.

3 Pour the batter into the prepared pan and bake in the oven for 50 minutes. Remove from the oven and cool in the pan on a wire rack for about 15 minutes. Serve warm or at room temperature.

Apple Crumble

At the Sivananda Yoga Centre in London, we have frequent dinners for students who are taking our Yoga Beginners' Course. On the fifth class they have a practical as well as theoretical introduction to "Proper Diet." This is our favorite quick-and-easy dessert. Serve it on its own or topped with Cornmeal Custard (page 114) or yogurt. Serves 8 to 12

Filling:
8 apples, sliced
⅔ cup raisins (optional)
1 teaspoon ground cinnamon
1 teaspoon lemon juice
½ teaspoon grated fresh gingerroot

Topping:
2½ cups rolled oats or Granola (page 26)
1¼ cups whole wheat flour
½ teaspoon salt
½ cup butter or margarine
1⅔ cups honey, corn and barley malt syrup,
  maple syrup, or date syrup

1 Heat the oven to 375°F. Butter an 8-inch square baking dish. Mix all the filling ingredients together and transfer to the dish.

2 To make the topping, combine the rolled oats or granola, flour, and salt. Melt the butter or margarine, add the honey or syrup, and mix well. Stir the liquid mixture into the oatmeal. Spoon the topping over the filling. Bake for about 50 minutes; the filling should be soft but not too runny.

• **Date-Banana Crumble:** For the filling, cook 9 ounces dates in 1 cup water for 10 minutes. Add 3 mashed ripe bananas and 2 tablespoons lemon juice. Add a scant 1 cup sweetened dried coconut, if desired. Cook for 5 minutes, then mash the ingredients, leaving the bananas slightly chunky. Make the topping and bake as for the main recipe.

• **Apricot-Fig Slice:** Place 12 ounces dried apricots and 12 ounces dried figs in a pan with 1 cup orange juice and 1 teaspoon grated orange zest. Cook over medium heat until soft, then transfer to a food processor or blender and blend until smooth. Spread two-thirds of the topping in the baking dish as a bottom. Spread the purée over it and sprinkle the remaining crumble mixture on top. Bake as for the main recipe.

Pumpkin Tart
A festive favorite at the New York center's Thanksgiving dinner. Serve the pie with whipped cream, or Tofu Whipped Dream or Toasted Nut Dream (both page 115). Makes two 8-inch pies

Filling:
1 medium pumpkin
7½ tablespoons maple syrup
4 ounces silken tofu
¼ teaspoon sea salt
½ teaspoon ground cinnamon
¼ teaspoon ground ginger
Pinch of ground mace or freshly grated nutmeg

Pinch of ground cloves
1 tablespoon soy flour
Pastry Dough:
2½ cups whole wheat pastry flour
1 teaspoon sea salt
4 tablespoons wheat germ or sesame seeds
⅔ cup plus 2 teaspoons corn oil
7 tablespoons chilled sparkling mineral water

1 Heat the oven to 375°F. Make the filling first. Cut the pumpkin into eighths and remove the seeds and stringy bits. Place the pumpkin in a baking tray, cover with foil, and bake in the oven for 45 to 60 minutes, until soft.

2 Meanwhile, make the dough. Sift the flour and salt into a large bowl. Stir in the wheat germ or sesame seeds. Blend in the oil until the pieces are the size of peas. Add the water, 1 tablespoon at a time, until the mixture is moist. Knead just enough to hold the dough together. Divide the dough in half and roll into two balls, wrap in waxed paper, and chill for 30 minutes.

3 Remove the pumpkin from the oven, peel it, and purée in a food processor or blender. Add the maple syrup and tofu and blend until smooth. Add the salt, spices, and soy flour and mix well.

4 Roll out the dough on a lightly floured surface, use to line two 8-inch tart pans with removeable bottoms, and prick with a fork. Bake in the oven for 8 to 10 minutes. Increase the temperature to 425°F. Divide the filling between the pastry shells and bake for 45 minutes, until the filling is set.

Tofu Cream Pie
This nourishing pie is the perfect dessert to follow a light main course. Decorate the pie with fresh seasonal fruit, if desired. Serves 8

Pastry dough:
3 tablespoons maple syrup
4 tablespoons oil
4 tablespoons water
1¾ cups rolled oats plus 1 tablespoon
6⅔ tablespoons whole wheat flour
½ cup sunflower seeds
Pinch of salt

Filling:
3 ounces soft tofu
1 to 2 tablespoons tahini
Grated zest of 1 lemon
⅓ cup plus 1 tablespoon maple syrup
4 tablespoons oil
4 tablespoons water
Pinch of salt

1 Heat the oven to 400°F and grease a 9-inch round springform pan.

2 To make the dough, whisk together the maple syrup, oil, and water. Add the rolled oats, flour, sunflower seeds, and salt; mix well. Pat the mixture onto the bottom and up the sides of the pan to a depth of about 1 inch. Bake in the oven for 10 to 15 minutes, until golden brown. Place the pan on a wire rack and leave to cool. Reduce the oven temperature to 350°F.

3 Put all the filling ingredients in a food processor or blender and purée until smooth. Pour into the baked crust. Bake for 25 to 30 minutes, until the filling is golden and set. Cool before serving.

Banana-Nut Tart
When this recipe was featured in our Yoga Life *magazine, it received rave reviews from readers. Bananas are especially beneficial for yoga practitioners, as they are said to increase humility and calmness.* Serves 8

Piecrust:
2½ cups rolled oats
1½ cups whole wheat flour
1 tablespoon honey or date syrup
⅔ cup oil
2⅓ cups sunflower seeds
Water for mixing

Filling:
1¼ cups cashew nuts
5 ounces pitted dates
4½ cups water
2 tablespoons arrowroot
1 teaspoon grated orange zest
1 teaspoon vanilla extract
2 bananas, plus slices for decoration
1¾ cups chopped walnuts

1 Heat the oven to 400°F. Grease a 9-inch loose-bottomed round tart pan. To make the piecrust, mix all the ingredients together, adding a little water to bind them.

2 Spread the mixture in the greased pan, using your hand to spread the mix evenly around the bottom and side of the pan. Bake in the oven for 10 to 15 minutes, until golden. Leave the pie shell to cool completely before removing from the pan.

3 To make the filling, put all the ingredients, except the bananas and chopped walnuts, in a food processor or blender and purée until smooth. Transfer the mixture to a pan and cook over low heat until thick. Remove from the heat and leave to cool.

4 Slice the 2 bananas into the pie shell. Pour the cooled filling on top and decorate with banana slices and the chopped nuts. Chill until set.

Sivananda Cookies
These large, energy-packed cookies are a standard after-class treat at most Sivanada Yoga centers around the world. They are very nutritious and make a meal in themselves. Makes 12

3 cups plus 1 tablespoon rolled oats
¾ cup plus 1 tablespoon whole wheat flour
¾ cup brown sugar
⅓ cup raisins or golden raisins
⅓ cup raw unsalted peanuts
1½ teaspoons ground cinnamon

1½ teaspoons ground ginger
½ teaspoon freshly grated nutmeg
½ teaspoon baking powder
¾ cup plus 2 tablespoons oil
About ¾ cup plus 2 tablespoons water

1 Heat the oven to 400°F. Grease two or three baking sheets. Combine the dry ingredients in a large mixing bowl, add the oil, and mix thoroughly. Stir in enough water to make a firm dough.

2 Take a spoonful of dough, about the size of a ping-pong ball. Roll it into a ball, place on one of the baking sheets, and flatten to a circle about 4 inches in diameter. Repeat to make 12 cookies. Bake in the oven for 12 to 15 minutes, until golden at the edges. Cool on a wire rack.

• Use sunflower seeds, roughly chopped almonds, and/or unsweetened dried coconut instead of, or as well as, the unsalted peanuts.

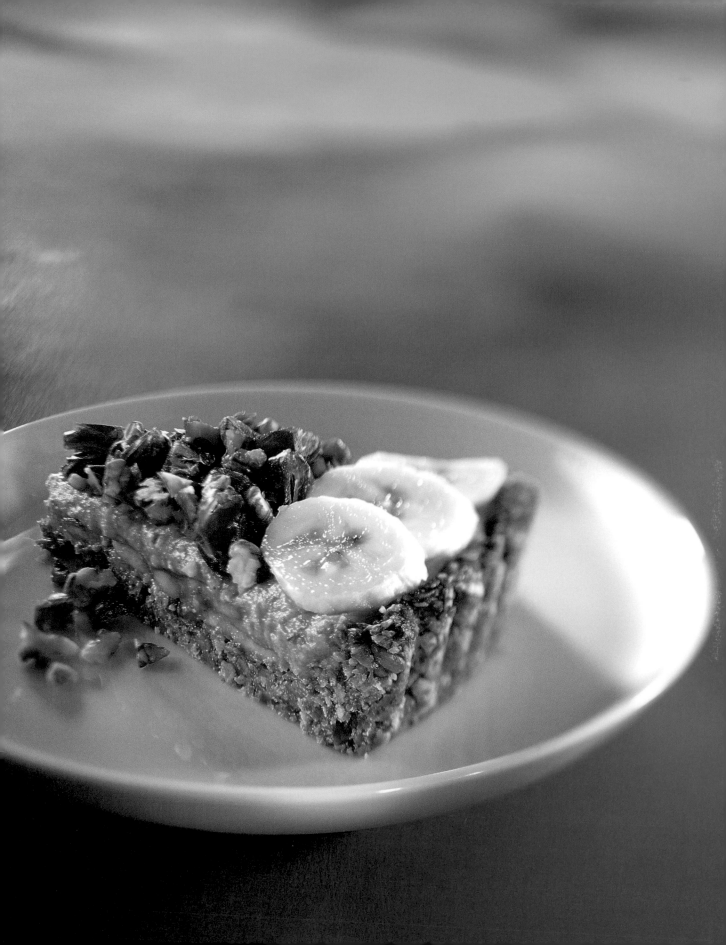

Gingerbread
The ginger in this warming traditional cake helps to stoke the digestive fire. Gingerbread can be served on its own, or spread with butter, jam, or Orange Butter Frosting (page 115), or served with Lemon Sauce (page 114).
Makes 16 squares

½ cup oil
7½ tablespoons molasses
¾ cup plus 2 tablespoons soy milk or
   plain yogurt
½ teaspoon salt

3¾ cups whole wheat flour
⅓ teaspoon ground cloves
1½ teaspoons baking soda
⅔ cup teaspoon ground ginger
1 teaspoon ground cinnamon

1 Heat the oven to 350°F. Lightly grease an 8-inch square cake pan.

2 Mix the oil, molasses, and soy milk or yogurt in a large mixing bowl. In a separate bowl, combine the dry ingredients and sift them into the molasses mixture, stirring in the bran from the sifter; mix thoroughly.

3 Pour Into the prepared pan and bake in the oven for 40 minutes. The cake is ready when a fine skewer inserted into the center comes out clean. Leave to cool in the pan. Turn out and cut into squares to serve.

Carob-Nut Brownies
Although it is often used as a chocolate substitute, carob has its own very distinctive taste. It has a very low-fat content and is rich in vitamins and minerals. These brownies may be served plain or iced with Carob Frosting (page 115). Makes 24

⅔ cup oil or butter, melted
¾ cup honey or date syrup
2¼ cups water
4 cups plus 1 tablespoon whole wheat flour
1¼ cups milk powder (page 104)

1⅔ cups carob powder
½ teaspoon salt
2 teaspoons baking powder
2¼ cups walnut pieces

1 Heat the oven to 350°F. Grease an 8- x 12-inch baking pan.

2 Mix the oil or butter, honey or date syrup, and water in a large mixing bowl. In a separate bowl, mix the flour, milk powder, carob powder, salt, and baking powder. Sift them into the honey mixture, stirring in the bran that remains in the sifter. The consistency should be fairly runny; add more water if necessary. Stir in the walnut pieces.

3 Pour the batter into the pan and bake in the oven for 30 minutes. Leave to cool in the pan, then turn out and cut into squares.

• **Wheat Germ Brownies:** Reduce the amount of honey or date syrup to 7½ tablespoons and add 2½ tablespoons molasses and 2 teaspoons vanilla extract. Omit the carob powder and reduce the quantity of walnut pieces to 1¾ cups. Stir 1 cup raisins and 3½ tablespoons lightly toasted wheat germ into the batter with the walnut pieces.

Applesauce Spice Cake

Cloves, cinnamon, and nutmeg give this cake a wonderful flavor, making it perfect for an afternoon snack or a festive cake at Christmastime. The cake can be served plain or covered with Butter Frosting (page 115). Serves 6 to 10

3 eating apples
½ cup water
5 tablespoons honey or barley malt syrup
4 tablespoons butter, melted, or oil
2½ cups whole wheat flour
1 teaspoon baking soda
½ teaspoon sea salt

1 teaspoon ground cinnamon
½ teaspoon ground cloves
½ teaspoon ground allspice
½ teaspoon freshly grated nutmeg
¼ teaspoon ground ginger
1 cup chopped nuts (untoasted and unsalted) or raisins

1 Heat the oven to 375°F. Grease and flour a 9- x 5-inch bread pan.

2 Peel the apples if they are not organic. Quarter them, remove the cores, and cut into thin slices. Place in a pan with the water, cover, and simmer over low heat for about 10 minutes, until the apples are soft. Remove from the heat and mash to a smooth sauce.

3 Mix the applesauce, honey or barley malt syrup, and melted butter or oil in a large mixing bowl until smooth. In a separate bowl, mix the flour, baking soda, salt, and spices, then sift into the applesauce mixture, stirring in the bran that remains in the sifter. Stir until blended; do not beat. Add the nuts or raisins. Pour into the bread pan and bake in the oven for 40 to 50 minutes, or until firm to the touch. Leave to cool in the pan before slicing and serving.

Peanut Butter-Carob Cake

Serves 8 to 10

Peanut butter batter:
6 tablespoons butter
1 cup less 1 tablespoon honey or other sweetener
2 teaspoons vanilla extract
½ cup plain yogurt
3 tablespoons milk
3 cups less 1 tablespoon whole wheat flour

2 teaspoons baking powder
Pinch of salt
½ cup plus 1½ tablespoons peanut butter
Carob batter:
2 tablespoons milk
½ teaspoon honey
1 tablespoon carob powder
¼ teaspoon ground cinnamon

1 Heat the oven to 375°F. Lightly grease an 8-inch square cake pan.

2 To make the peanut butter batter, cream the butter and honey or other sweetener in a large mixing bowl, then add the vanilla extract, yogurt, and milk and mix well. Sift the flour, baking powder, and salt into the butter mixture, stirring in the bran that remains in the sifter; stir well. Transfer 1 cup of this batter to a separate bowl; set aside for the carob mixture. Stir the peanut butter into the remaining batter and spoon it into the prepared cake pan.

3 To make the carob batter, add the milk, honey, carob powder, and cinnamon to the reserved batter. Stir the carob batter into the cake batter in the pan in a zigzag pattern. Level the surface and bake in the oven for about 30 minutes, until firm to the touch. Cool in the pan for a few minutes, cut into squares, and serve warm or cool.

Tofu-Prune Cake
When we tested this recipe at our London center, the demand for copies of the recipe reached an all-time high. Dates or other dried fruits may be substituted for the prunes. Serve with fresh fruit, if desired. Serves 12

1 cup oil
1 pound firm tofu
1½ cups packed brown sugar
Finely grated zest and juice of 2 lemons

4¾ cups sifted self-rising flour
1 teaspoon baking powder
4½ cups chopped prunes
Orange or Lemon Butter Frosting (page 115)

1 Heat the oven to 350°F. Grease a 9½-inch round cake pan and line the bottom with baking parchment.

2 Put the oil, tofu, sugar, and lemon juice in a food processor or blender and blend until creamy and smooth. Transfer to a mixing bowl and sift in the flour and baking powder. Stir in the lemon zest and prunes.

3 Spoon the batter into the prepared cake pan and bake in the oven for 1 to 1¼ hours, until a fine skewer inserted into the center comes out clean. Leave to cool in the pan, then turn out and spread with frosting before serving.

Passion Cake
This cake is a favorite at our Easter retreats. We take over a large country house and immerse ourselves in yoga practice for five days, with periodic breaks for a game of football, a talent show, or a bit of sweetness such as this cake. Serves 8 to 12

2 cups plus 1 tablespoon whole wheat flour
2 teaspoons baking powder
1 teaspoon apple-pie spice
2 teaspoons ground cinnamon
3 tablespoons soy flour
6 tablespoons water
1¼ cups packed brown sugar
½ cup chopped pecans or walnuts
1 large very ripe banana
⅓ cup chopped dried figs
2 tablespoons golden raisins

1 tablespoon lime marmalade
1⅓ cups finely grated carrots
¾ cup oil
Frosting:
7 ounces creamed coconut (look for this in
   health-food stores and Asian food stores)
About 6 tablespoons hot water
Grated zest of ½ orange
3 to 4 tablespoons confectioners' sugar
3 tablespoons orange juice
Scant 1 cup sweetened dried coconut, toasted

1 Heat the oven to 375°F. Grease and line the bottom of an 8-inch round cake pan. Combine the whole wheat flour, baking powder, and spices in a large mixing bowl. Mix the soy flour with the water and stir into the bowl with the sugar and nuts. Mash the banana and add it with the figs, golden raisins, marmalade, carrots, and oil; mix thoroughly.

2 Transfer the batter to the prepared pan and level the top. Bake in the oven for 40 to 50 minutes, or until firm to the touch. Leave to cool in the pan. Using a round-bladed knife, ease the sides of the cake away from the pan, then carefully turn out and peel off the lining paper.

3 To make the frosting, mash the creamed coconut in a bowl with some of the hot water, using a fork, then beat in the orange zest, confectioners' sugar, and orange juice with enough hot water to make a smooth consistency for spreading on the top and side of the cake. Sprinkle evenly with the toasted coconut.

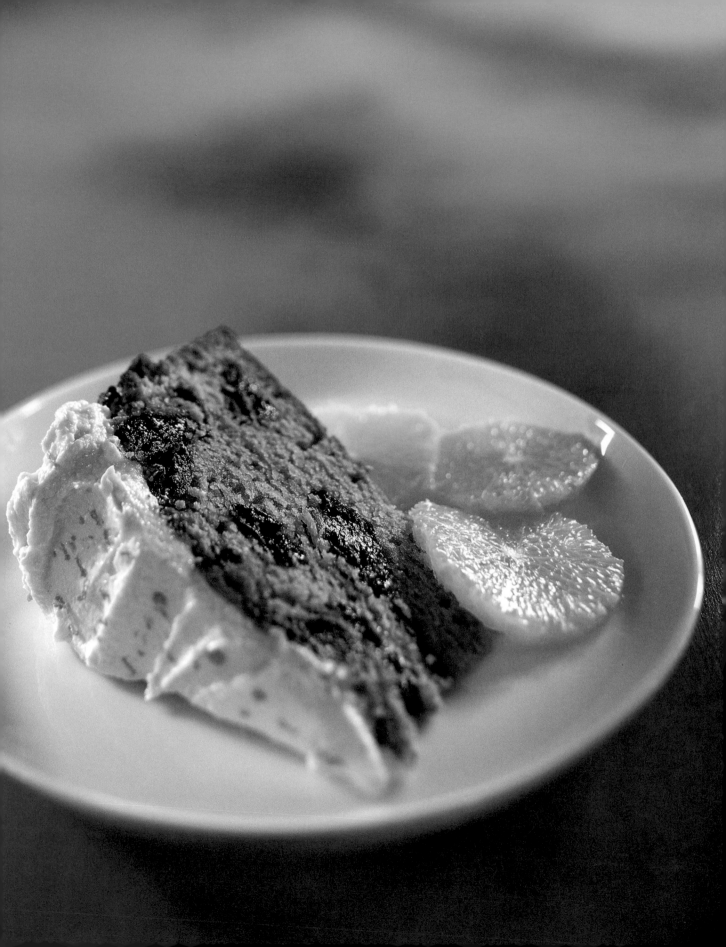

Rich Tofu Fruitcake

No baking powder is needed for Nigel Walker's scrumptious cake because the tofu and bread crumbs make this light. Creamed coconut is available from Asian and health-food stores. Serves 8 to 12

1 orange
½ lemon
3½ cups fresh whole wheat bread crumbs
1¾ cups currants
1 cup golden raisins
1 tablespoon mugi miso
4 tablespoons apple juice concentrate
2 tablespoons whole wheat flour
9 ounces tofu, mashed
3 tablespoons barley malt syrup

2 eating apples, grated
1¼ cups walnuts, lightly toasted
2 tablespoons cold-pressed corn oil
Scant 1 cup rolled oats
Orange juice (optional)
1 teaspoon freshly grated nutmeg
3 teaspoons ground cinnamon
2 teaspoons ground ginger
4 ounces creamed coconut, shredded and dissolved in 1¼ cups water

1 Heat the oven to 325°F. Line a 9-inch cake pan with parchment paper and oil it. Peel the orange and lemon. Slice the peel finely. Chop the flesh, removing the pips.

2 Stir all the ingredients with a wooden spoon, adding more juice or oats to achieve a consistency like thick, wet mud. Spoon into the cake pan, cover with foil, and bake in the oven for 3 hours, or until firm to the touch. Leave to cool on a wire rack for several hours before turning out.

Cornmeal Custard Serves 4

4½ cups milk or soy milk
2 tablespoons honey or maple syrup
Handful of golden raisins (optional)

½ teaspoon vanilla extract
3 tablespoons yellow cornmeal

Place the milk, honey or maple syrup, golden raisins, and vanilla extract in a pan and bring to a boil. Whisk in the cornmeal slowly and cook until the custard thickens, whisking frequently. Serve hot.

Ginger and Lemon Sauce

Omit the ground ginger to make a tangy lemon sauce. Serves 4

Grated zest and juice of ½ lemon
4 tablespoons apple juice

2 tablespoons turbinado sugar
½ teaspoon ground ginger

Mix all the ingredients in a pan and bring to a boil slowly, stirring constantly. Simmer for about 5 minutes, then serve hot.

Raisin Sauce Serves 4

1⅓ cups raisins
1¼ to 1¾ cups water

About 1 teaspoon vanilla extract
About 1 teaspoon ground cinnamon

Put the raisins in a pan with enough of the water to cover them. Bring to a boil, lower the heat, and simmer for 20 minutes. Transfer to a blender and blend to a coarse or a smooth purée. If it is too thick, add more water. Add vanilla extract and cinnamon to taste. Reheat hot or warm.

Raspberry Sauce *Raspberries are said to enhance kindness. If you like, strawberries can be used instead; they may not need sweetening.* Serves 4

5 ounces fresh raspberries

About 2 tablespoons honey or brown sugar

Purée the raspberries in a food processor or blender. Add honey or brown sugar to taste and serve hot.

Butter Frosting *Use whole milk powder, available from Indian stores and health-food stores.* Enough for one cake

1 cup butter, at room temperature
1/3 cup honey or other sweetener
2 tablespoons milk

1/2 tablespoon vanilla extract
1 3/4 cups cups whole milk powder (page 104)

Whip the butter in a food processor or blender. Add the remaining ingredients, one at a time, beating after each addition. Leave to cool before using.

• **Lemon or Orange Butter Frosting:** Omit the milk and vanilla extract and add the juice of 2 lemons or 3 oranges. Sprinkle with a little grated zest, if desired.
• **Carob Frosting:** Use 1/2 cup milk powder and add 1/2 cup carob powder.

Tofu Whipped Dream *Suitable for vegans, this dreamy topping can be used as a cake frosting or on desserts.* Serves 4 to 6

8 ounces tofu, steamed for 2 to 3 minutes
3 tablespoons honey, maple syrup, or apple juice concentrate

1 teaspoon vanilla extract
Water or fruit juice, if necessary

Place the tofu, honey, maple syrup, or apple juice concentrate and vanilla extract in a food processor or blender and blend until the mixture is like whipped cream. Add water or fruit juice to thin it, if desired. Use straight away or chill overnight before serving.

• Use rose water or orange flower-water instead of vanilla extract.
• Add the grated zest of 1 orange or lemon.
• Add 2 tablespoons finely ground almonds and a few drops of almond extract.

Toasted Nut Dream *Serve this nut cream as a topping for fruit salads, pies, or any other desserts.* Serves 4 to 6

3/4 cup plus 1 tablespoon hazelnuts
2/3 cup soy milk
1 teaspoon lemon juice

1 to 2 tablespoons honey
Pinch of salt

Toast the hazelnuts in a hot, dry skillet over high heat until lightly brown; leave to cool. Put all the ingredients in a food processor or blender and blend until creamy.

• Substitute almonds for the hazelnuts and add a few drops of vanilla extract.
• Substitute walnuts for the hazelnuts and use maple syrup instead of honey.

FINISHING
TOUCHES

"Serve, Love, Give, Purify,
Meditate, Realize."

Swami Sivananda

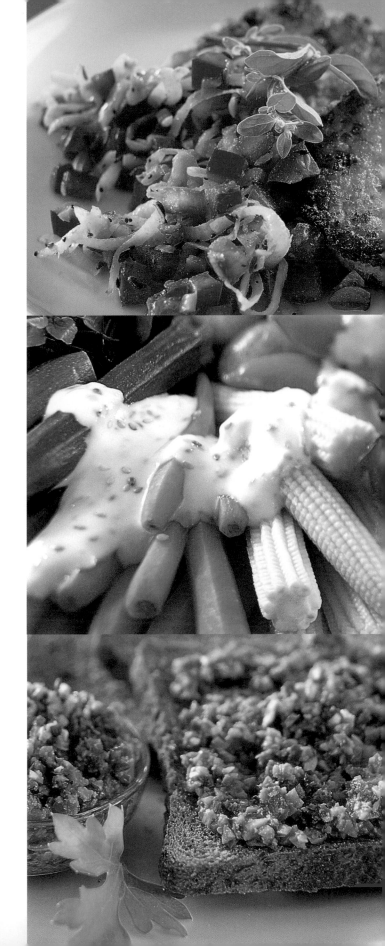

Traditionally it is suggested that food be offered with love to all guests, even if they have arrived uninvited. The wise person graciously receives any guest with the words "Food is ready." The best food should be given in abundance with faith and devotion, courtesy, and humility. Then the yogic principle that "the guest is GOD" will become a living, breathing reality.

Through this practice of service, love for humanity develops. From love, one learns to give of oneself. Only then are we able to purify the mind completely and prepare it to meditate and realize the peace and happiness that lie within.

While most vegetables, grains, and proteins taste good by themselves, a simple sauce or salad dressing can help to light the digestive fire. It is this digestive fire that "cooks" the food within the body, transforming it into blood, flesh, and bone. Adding a finishing touch such as a dressing or sauce can turn a simple dish into a special meal.

Seed Toppings   Seed toppings make a lovely garnish to sprinkle over salads, vegetables, beans, or grains. Seeds can be rinsed before toasting, if desired; it makes them expand and helps to prevent them from burning.

Pumpkin Seed and Wakame Topping: Heat the oven to 350°F. Toast a handful of pumpkin seeds in a dry skillet over high heat until they "pop." Place 4 or 5 strips of wakame on a baking sheet and bake in the oven for 5 to 10 minutes, until dry. Grind the seaweed and pumpkin seeds together, making the mixture as coarse or as fine as you like.

Tamari and Sunflower Seeds: Toast a handful of sunflower seeds in a hot, dry skillet over high heat until they are golden. Turn off the heat and add a few drops of tamari to coat the seeds.

Gomasio: This is a tasty way to reduce salt consumption. Toast a handful of sesame seeds in a hot, dry skillet over high heat until they give off a pleasant aroma. Combine 1 part kosher salt or coarse sea salt to 15 parts sesame seeds and grind with a mortar and pestle. It is worth making a large amount of this mixture at a time as it stores well.

Basic Salad Dressing   *There is no limit to the ingredients that can be used in salad dressings, but as vinegar is not used in a yogic diet dressings are usually made with fresh citrus juices. Freshly squeezed grapefruit is the least acid-forming of all citrus fruits and makes a refreshing change from lemon. Or, try orange juice instead of, or in combination with, the lemon juice. Try to use cold-pressed oils. Olive oil is always a treat in a salad dressing; use it alone or in combination with other oils. Yogurt, tofu, and lecithin are expanders and are used to give dressings a creamy texture. Tofu should be steamed for 2 to 3 minutes before using it in the dressings. Use any herbs you wish, such as basil, rosemary, thyme, mint, or dill, or seeds such as caraway or cumin. Some people also like to blend in 1 tablespoon honey. At the Sivananda Yoga Retreat in the Bahamas, we often blend the salad left from the previous meal with a little lemon juice, tamari, and dill or other herbs. It never comes out the same twice, is always good, and guests beg for the "special green salad dressing" recipe.*   Serves 4 to 6

½ cup oil
4 tablespoons lemon juice

1 tablespoon tamari, or 1 teaspoon sea salt

Place all the ingredients in a bowl or screw-top jar and whisk together or shake until mixed.

• **French Dressing:** Use salt not tamari. Blend the ingredients in a blender with 2 chopped tomatoes, 1 tablespoon fresh dill or ½ teaspoon dried dillweed, and ¼ teaspoon pepper.

• Add any chopped fresh herbs or seeds such as caraway or cumin.

• Use freshly squeezed grapefruit or orange juice instead of the lemon juice (or a mixture of all three).

Sunflower Seed Dressing *This is the current favorite at the London center. Sunflower seeds, which are rich in B vitamins, give a creaminess to this dressing and stop the other ingredients from separating.* Serves 4 to 6

5 tablespoons oil
2 tablespoons lemon juice
⅔ cup sunflower seeds

1 tablespoon tamari, or 1 teaspoon salt
5 tablespoons water

Put all the ingredients in a blender and blend until smooth. Add more water or more sunflower seeds, depending on how thick you want the dressing to be.

• Use toasted sesame seed oil and add a ½-inch piece of fresh gingerroot, peeled and grated.
• Replace the sunflower seeds with pumpkin seeds, or use a mixture of the two.

Tahini-Mint Dressing *The tahini gives this dressing a hint of Middle Eastern flavors. It is particularly good drizzled over salad leaves or fruit. Tahini has a very high oil content, so no extra oil is needed.* Makes about 1 cup

6 tablespoons tahini
Juice of 1 lemon
Dash of tamari

½ cup water
1 tablespoon chopped fresh mint

Mix all the ingredients together in a blender or whisk them in a bowl. Thin the dressing with a little more water, if necessary.

• Use 3 tablespoons peanut butter instead of tahini and omit the mint.
• For a lovely topping for fruit salads, omit the tamari and use apple juice instead of water. Add a little honey, if desired.
• Omit the water and serve it as a party dip with vegetable crudités, crisps, or crackers.

Creamy Italian Dressing *This rich, thick creamy dressing is excellent for salads. Alternatively, it can be used as a dressing for pasta.* Serves 4 to 6

½ cup chick-peas, cooked
6 tablespoons olive oil
1 teaspoon dried oregano
Pinch of dried dillweed

3 tablespoons lemon juice
1 teaspoon salt
½ teaspoon pepper

Put the chick-peas in a food processor or blender and blend until smooth. Add all the remaining ingredients and blend again until smooth. If necessary, thin with water or more oil to the desired consistency. Chill before serving.

Seeded Yogurt Dressing
Caraway seeds—excellent for helping the digestion—give this oil-free dressing a sweet-and-spicy taste. Fennel, anise, or cumin seeds can be used instead of caraway. Makes about 1 cup

2 tablespoons sesame seeds
1 teaspoon caraway seeds
3/4 cup plus 2 tablespoons plain yogurt

1/2 teaspoon mustard powder
1 tablespoon lemon juice
1/2 teaspoon salt

Toast the seeds in a hot, dry skillet over high heat until they begin to smell aromatic. Crush them slightly and blend with the other ingredients in a blender or whisk them in a bowl. Thin with a little water, if necessary.

• For a richer dressing, substitute sour cream for all or part of the yogurt.
• For a vegan version, replace the yogurt with 7 ounces silken tofu, steamed for 2 to 3 minutes and crumbled.

Eggless Mayonnaise
Use as a healthy alternative to commercial mayonnaise. The lecithin is used as an emulsifier instead of eggs, but you can make it without, if preferred. Makes about 1 cup

2/3 cup soy milk
6 tablespoons oil
2 tablespoons lemon juice
1/2 teaspoon salt or tamari

1/4 teaspoon mustard powder
1 tablespoon liquid lecithin or 1 teaspoon
    lecithin granules (optional)

Place all the ingredients in a blender and blend until smooth. Leave the mayonnaise to set for about 1 hour before using.

• Add 1/2 teaspoon curry powder and 1/4 teaspoon turmeric.
• Add 1/2 bunch of finely chopped parsley.
• Blend in 2 tablespoons tahini.
• For a thicker mayonnaise, reduce the oil to 2 tablespoons and blend in 5 ounces tofu, steamed for 2 to 3 minutes and crumbled.
• For dill mayonnaise, mix in a small bunch of fresh dill, chopped, or 1 teaspoon dried dillweed, and 1 tablespoon tomato paste or 2 chopped tomatoes.

Cashew Gravy
With their high protein and mineral content, cashew nuts add a creamy richness to steamed vegetables or grains, increasing the nutritional value of a meal. Walnuts can be substituted, if preferred. Serves 6

1/3 cup raw cashews
1 tablespoon arrowroot

3/4 cup plus 2 tablespoons vegetable stock
    or water, plus extra if necessary
1 teaspoon tamari

Toast the cashews in a hot, dry skillet over high heat until lightly brown. Put the nuts, arrowroot, and stock or water in a food processor or blender and blend until smooth. Pour into a pan and heat over medium heat for 3 to 5 minutes, until thick, stirring constantly. Dilute with additional vegetable stock or water, if desired. Stir in the tamari and serve hot.

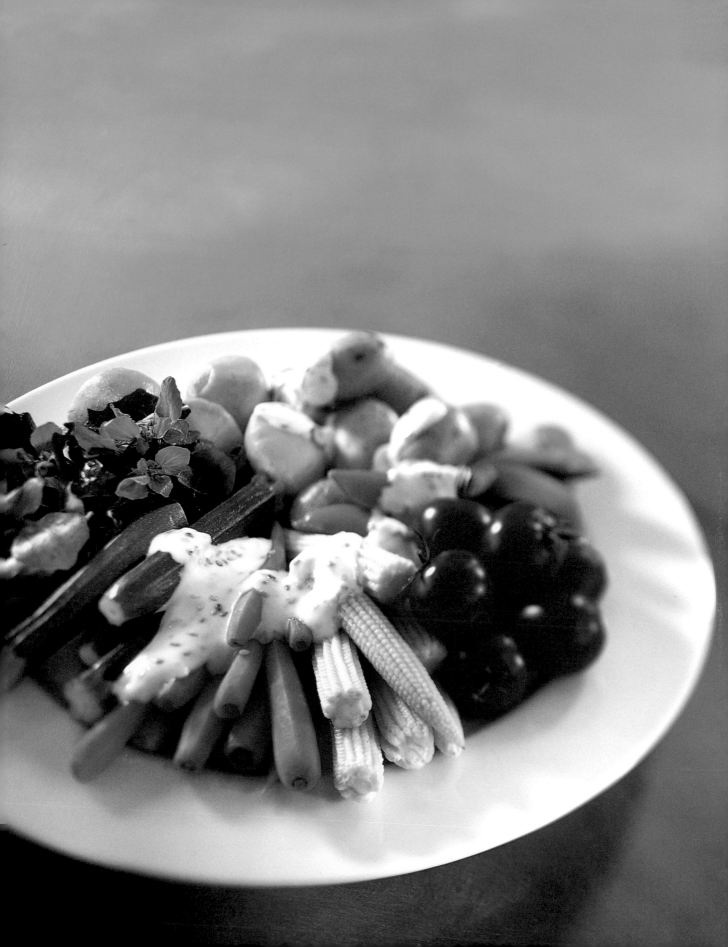

Rich Brown Gravy
Butter or margarine will give the best flavor but corn, safflower, or other low-cholesterol oils can be used. Any herbs, fresh or dried, can be added to this gravy: basil is especially suggested; sage, thyme, and savory will give a very traditional gravy; oregano, marjoram, or rosemary, a more Italian flavor. Whole wheat flour or chick-pea flour (also known as besan or gram flour) can be used instead of arrowroot. Chick-pea flour adds a lovely nutty flavor. Makes about 1½ cups

2 tablespoons butter or margarine
3 tablespoons arrowroot
1¼ cups water
Chopped fresh herbs or dried herbs to taste

2 tablespoons tamari
1 teaspoon tomato paste (optional)
Pepper to taste

Melt the butter or margarine in a pan over medium heat. Stir in the arrowroot and gradually whisk in the water, stirring continuously for a smooth, lumpfree sauce. If using dried herbs, add them with the water. Bring to simmering point and simmer until the gravy is thick. Add the tamari and tomato paste and fresh herbs, if using. Season with pepper.

• For a vegetable gravy, sauté about 1 cup grated vegetables (turnip, cabbage, and/or carrots) in the butter or margarine before adding the arrowroot. To give the gravy extra "zing," add 1 tablespoon grated fresh gingerroot. This is particularly good served with Kasha Varnishkas (page 62) or other grain dishes.
• Replace 4 tablespoons of the water with unsweetened apple or grape juice and add 1 teaspoon lemon juice just before serving.
• Omit the tomato paste and add 2 teaspoons nutritional yeast flakes, a pinch of dried sage and thyme, and 2 tablespoons lemon juice.
• Remove from the heat and stir in ½ cup grated vegetarian cheese, or 2 tablespoons miso, or ½ cup tahini.
• Add a pinch of ground cumin or paprika for a more piquant gravy.

Miso-Sesame Sauce
Miso is rich in vitamin B12 and has a warming and toning effect on the system, while sesame seeds are rich in calcium. Serve this sauce over steamed kale or other green vegetables for a balanced, appetizing dish. Serves 4

⅔ cup butter or margarine
Scant 1 cup sesame seeds

2 teaspoons white miso

Melt the butter or margarine in a small pan. Toast the sesame seeds in a hot, dry skillet over high heat until golden brown, stirring constantly to prevent them from burning. Remove from the heat. Add them to the melted butter and stir in the miso. Serve at once.

• Add 1 to 2 tablespoons chopped fresh parsley or cilantro to the melted butter and sauté briefly before adding the sesame seeds.
• Use half butter and half sesame oil.
• Add 1 teaspoon tamari with the miso.

No-Cheese Sauce *This is a vegan delight over steamed vegetables, grains, or legumes.* Serves 6 to 8

5 tablespoons margarine
½ cup whole wheat flour
3⅓ cups soy milk
½ teaspoon mustard powder

½ ounce nutritional yeast flakes
¼ teaspoon freshly grated nutmeg (optional)
Salt and pepper

Melt the margarine in a pan. Add the flour and cook over low heat for 1 to 2 minutes. Whisk in the soy milk and cook until thick. Add the mustard, yeast flakes, and nutmeg, if using. Season to taste with salt and pepper.

Tomato Sauce *This thick, chunky sauce can be served on vegetables, pasta, or grains. If possible, use deep red, juicy tomatoes and make the sauce in advance so it can stand for a few hours to bring out the flavor.* Makes about 2¼ cups

2 tablespoons olive oil
2 sticks of celery, finely chopped
1 carrot, grated
1 bay leaf
2½ cups fresh or canned tomatoes

⅔ cup tomato paste
2 tablespoons chopped fresh oregano or basil,
  or 1 tablespoon Italian seasoning
1 teaspoon salt
Pinch of pepper

Heat the oil in a skillet and sauté the celery over medium heat until soft. Add the carrot, bay leaf, tomatoes, and tomato paste and simmer for 45 minutes. Add the herbs and season with salt and pepper. Serve as a chunky sauce or purée in a food processor or blender for smooth sauce.

• To use in lasagne, substitute 1 pound mixed diced vegetables (zucchini, green bell pepper, carrot) for the celery and carrot.
• To use as a pizza topping, substitute for the celery 2½ cups yellow, and/or green bell peppers, cored, seeded and chopped. Add a pinch of cayenne pepper, if desired.

Ginger Sauce *A light, spicy sauce for steamed vegetables, noodles, or tofu. The healing properties of ginger are legion, and it plays a very strong part in the yogic diet, because it stimulates the digestion without having a similarly stimulating effect on the mind. It is excellent for warming the system, improving blood circulation, and helping to cure colds and flu.* Serves 4

¾ cup plus 2 tablespoons water
2 tablespoons tamari
2½ tablespoons molasses or barley malt syrup
1½ teaspoons cornstarch or arrowroot

1½ tablespoons water
1 teaspoon grated fresh gingerroot
1 tablespoon apple juice or white grape juice
2 teaspoons lemon juice

1 Heat the water in a pan. Add the tamari and the molasses or barley malt syrup and simmer over medium heat for about 5 minutes, stirring occasionally.

2 Dissolve the cornstarch or arrowroot in the 1½ tablespoons water. Add to the pan and bring to a boil. Add the grated ginger and apple or grape juice and cook for 2 minutes longer. Remove from the heat and stir in the lemon juice.

Salsa *This quick party dip is lightly spiced and perfect for serving with crudités, whole wheat crackers, or pita bread.* Serves 6

1 tablespoon oil
½ teaspoon celery seeds
1 teaspoon cumin seeds
1 small turnip, grated
1 fresh green chili, seeded and chopped
3½ cups finely chopped fresh tomatoes,

½ teaspoon ground coriander
½ teaspoon cayenne pepper
1 tablespoon chopped fresh oregano or
  ½ teaspoon dried oregano
1 teaspoon salt

Heat the oil in a heavy pan and toast the celery and cumin seeds over high heat until they "pop." Add the turnip and chili and sauté over medium heat for 5 minutes. Transfer to a food processor or blender and purée until smooth. Pour into a bowl and stir in the chopped tomatoes, spices, oregano, and salt. Leave to set and serve at room temperature.

Orange-Dill Sauce *The lime and ginger give this sauce a tang, making it a refreshing topping for steamed vegetables.* Serves 4 to 6

¾-inch piece fresh gingerroot, peeled and
  chopped
Grated zest and juice of 1 orange
Grated zest and juice of 1 lime
1 teaspoon salt
Pepper

¾ cup plus 2 tablespoons water
2 tablespoons arrowroot
2 tablespoons finely chopped fresh dill or
  1 tablespoon dried dillweed
3 tablespoons butter or margarine

1 Put all the ingredients, except the dill and butter or margarine, in a food processor or blender and blend until smooth. Stir in the dill.

2 Melt the butter or margarine in a pan, add the other ingredients, and cook over medium heat for 3 to 4 minutes until slightly thicker. Serve warm.

Gado-Gado *This traditional Indonesian sauce adds a piquant flavor to the simplest of dishes, such as lightly steamed carrots, green beans, asparagus, broccoli, and cauliflower, or grains. Use good-quality peanut butter.* Serves 4 to 6

1½ tablespoons oil
½ stick of celery, or ¼ green bell pepper,
  cored, seeded, and diced
1 tablespoon chopped fresh gingerroot
Pinch of curry powder, ground cumin, or
  cayenne pepper (optional)

⅔ cup crunchy peanut butter
About 1 cup boiling water
½ cup unsweetened dried coconut
2 tablespoons tamari
1½ teaspoons honey
Juice of ½ lemon

1 Heat the oil in a wok or skillet. Add the diced celery or green bell pepper, ginger, and curry powder, cumin, or cayenne pepper, if using. Sauté over low heat for about 5 minutes, until soft. Add the peanut butter, stirring to prevent it from scorching. When the mixture is bubbling, stir in enough boiling water to give it the consistency of thin cream.

2 Bring back to a boil over high heat. Lower the heat and add the coconut and tamari. Simmer for about 10 minutes, until the oil rises to the top of the sauce. Remove from the heat and stir in the honey and lemon juice.

Cranberry Sauce
High in vitamin C, the tart flavor of cranberries makes them the ideal accompaniment to rich dishes. This sauce is one of the traditions of Thanksgiving or Christmas dinner, but can be served at any time. Serves 4 to 6

¾ cup chopped dried dates	5 cloves
4 tablespoons water	½ orange, thinly sliced with the zest on
4 cups raw cranberries	4 tablespoons honey
2 cinnamon sticks, each 1 inch long	

1 Place the dates in a pan with the water. Bring to a boil, then remove from the heat and leave to stand for an hour or so.

2 Place the cranberries in a heavy pan with the cinnamon, cloves, orange slices, dates, and the water. Cook, uncovered, over medium heat until thick, then remove from the heat and leave to cool. Add the honey and leave to set before serving.

Coconut Chutney
This chutney is simple to prepare. Its spicy tang is cooled by the coconut, making it a suitable accompaniment for any meal. In South India, it is traditionally served with Dosas (page 28) for breakfast. Add a bunch of chopped fresh cilantro for a green chutney. Serves 4 to 6

Scant 1 cup unsweetened dried coconut	1 tablespoon ghee
3 tablespoons chopped curry leaves	1 teaspoon black mustard seeds
1 green chili, seeded and chopped	1 tablespoon lemon juice
½-inch piece fresh gingerroot, peeled and grated	1 to 2 teaspoons paprika
1 carrot, grated	1 teaspoon salt

1 Soak the coconut in just enough water to cover for 15 to 20 minutes, then squeeze out the liquid. Add the chopped curry leaves, green chilli, ginger, and carrot. Toss the mixture with your hands until everything is well mixed.

2 Heat the ghee in a skillet and toast the mustard seeds over high heat until they "pop." Add the ghee and mustard seeds to the coconut mixture and mix well, then stir in the lemon juice, paprika, and salt.

Mint Chutney
A traditional accompaniment for Indian snacks. Try it with any type of savory dish or spread on sandwiches. Serves 4 to 6

4 to 6 cashew nuts	1 tablespoon chopped fresh mint
1½-inch piece of fresh gingerroot, peeled and grated	1 teaspoon lemon juice
1 green bell pepper, cored, seeded, and chopped (optional)	1 teaspoon salt
	½ teaspoon ground coriander
	4 tablespoons plain yogurt (optional)

Put the cashew nuts, ginger, green bell pepper, if using, and mint in a food processor or blender and blend to a fine pulp. Add the rest of the ingredients and mix thoroughly. Leave the chutney to set for at least 1 hour before serving.

Miso-Nut Spread
This is a healthy, yeast-free alternative to the commercial yeast extract spreads. It can be used as a topping or as a spread on bread or crackers. Add a little salad for an unusual sandwich filling. Serves 4 to 6

2 tablespoons hazelnuts or almonds
2 tablespoons light miso

1 tablespoon water

Toast the nuts in a hot, dry skillet over high heat until lightly brown. Place them in a blender with the miso and water. Blend together until smooth.

• Substitute any nut butter or tahini for the nuts.
• Vary the type of miso.

Olive Spread
This attractive spread serves four as a sandwich stuffing or many more as a topping on crackers for party nibbles. Spread on whole wheat bread and garnished with salad cress or parsley sprigs, it makes a tasty picnic or lunch snack. Serves 4 to 6

20 green olives stuffed with pimento
3 tablespoons walnut pieces

½ red bell pepper, cored, seeded, and chopped
2 tablespoons oil

Put all the ingredients in a blender and blend to a coarse purée. Alternatively, chop the ingredients very finely. Leave to set for about 1 hour before serving.

• For a green spread, omit the walnuts and pepper. Halve the amount of oil and blend in 4 tablespoons chopped fresh parsley and 2 tablespoons tahini.

Cottage Cheese Topping
This makes a flavorful topping for steamed vegetables and new or baked potatoes, or it can be spread on toast for a nutritious breakfast or a light lunch dish. Serves 4 to 6

1 teaspoon lemon juice
1 tablespoon raw wheat germ
3 tablespoons cottage cheese

1 tablespoon seasame oil
1 cup plain yogurt or sour cream

Mix all the ingredients together in a bowl and serve straight away.

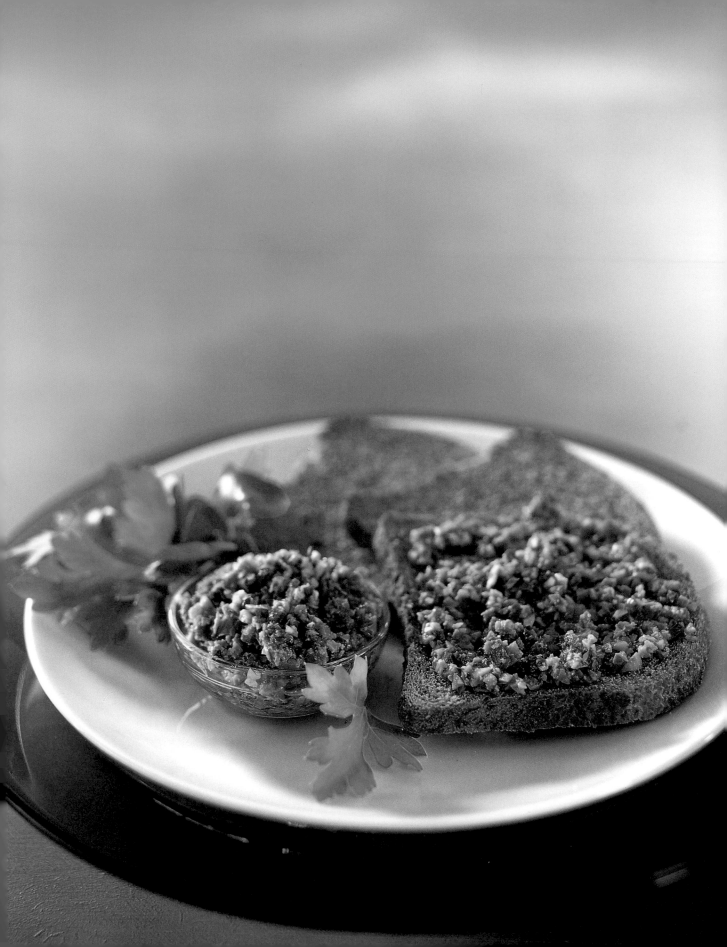

YOGIC
FEASTS

"You are an ocean of Bliss, an embodiment of Joy. You are in reality the Lord of the three worlds. If you give up egoism, selfishness, and greed, you will realize God here and now. God has given you faculties and potentialities, so rise up. Keep your faculties bright and brilliant by taking a pure diet."

Swami Sivananda

OM
Anna Poorne Sadha Poorne
Shankara Prana Vallabhe
Jnana Vairagya Siddyartham
Bhiksham Dhehee Cha Parvati

Divine Mother, who comes to out table as food,
You are the endlessly bountiful, benefactress of all.
Please grant us wisdom, dispassion, strength, and
O Mother, give us health.

OM
Mata Me Parvati Devi
Pita Devo Mahashwara
Bandhava Siva Bhaktascha
Swadesho Bhuvana Trayam

Mother Nature is my Mother Divine
The Lord of the Universe is my Father
All the people of the world are my friends and relatives.
The entire universe is my home.

Sankaracharya,

Annapoorneshwari Stotran, 11-12

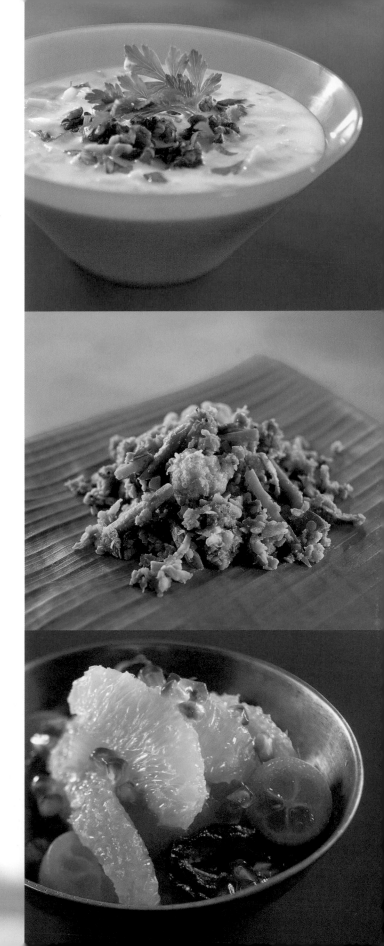

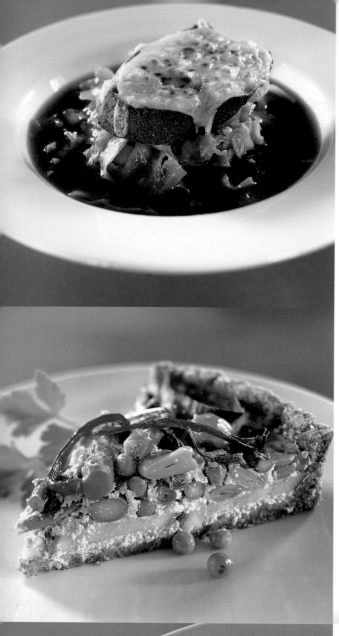

April in Paris

Potage Choux au Gratin
Tofu Quiche
Pommes de Terre Roti au Romarin
Petits Pois à la Français
Prune Mousse

Serves 4 to 6

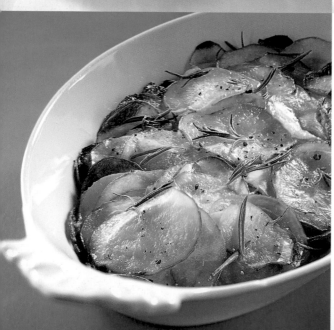

Any lunch shared with family and friends can be a joyous occasion. This simple, yet elegant menu sparkles with the rejuvenating lightness of a Paris spring.

Top left—Potage Choux au Gratin: A sattvic variation on the traditional onion soup theme.

Center left—The Tofu Quiche: Another one of Nigel Walker's delightful recipes. Nigel (aka Nagaraj) is a trained Cordon Bleu chef, former staff member of the Sivananda Yoga centers, and a leading macrobiotic chef and cooking teacher in Britain. The quiche can be made slightly ahead and served warm or cool.

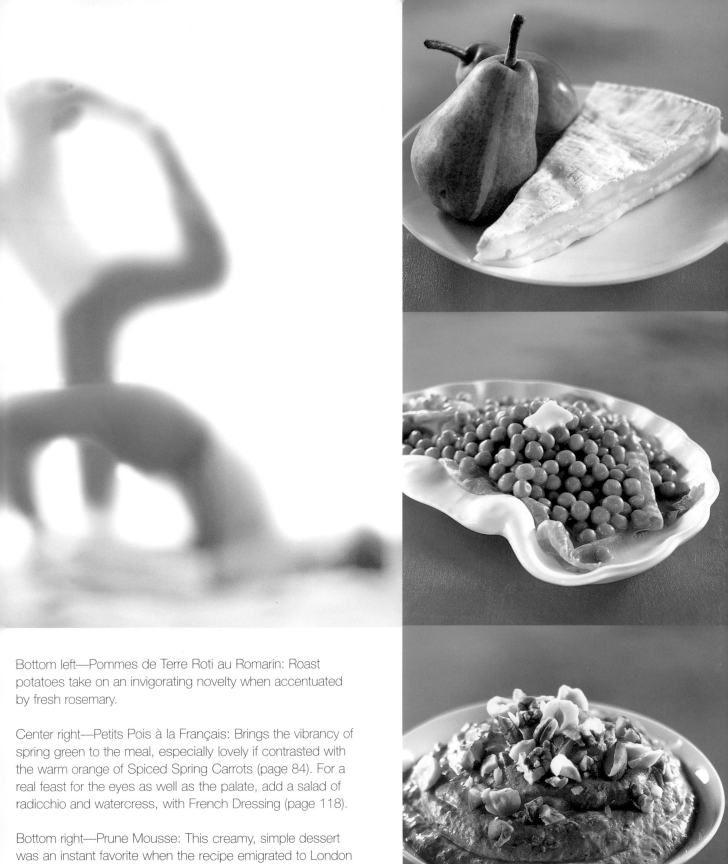

Bottom left—Pommes de Terre Roti au Romarin: Roast potatoes take on an invigorating novelty when accentuated by fresh rosemary.

Center right—Petits Pois à la Français: Brings the vibrancy of spring green to the meal, especially lovely if contrasted with the warm orange of Spiced Spring Carrots (page 84). For a real feast for the eyes as well as the palate, add a salad of radicchio and watercress, with French Dressing (page 118).

Bottom right—Prune Mousse: This creamy, simple dessert was an instant favorite when the recipe emigrated to London from the Sivananda Yoga Center in Paris.

Potage Choux au Gratin

2 to 4 tablespoons butter or margarine
1 white cabbage, coarsely shredded
1¾ quarts water
3 bay leaves

½ cup tamari
1 French bread (whole wheat, if possible)
2½ cups grated vegetarian cheese

1 Melt the butter or margarine in a pan and sauté the cabbage over medium heat for about 15 minutes, until soft and translucent, stirring occasionally.

2 Bring the water to the boil. Add the sautéed cabbage and bay leaves, cover, and simmer for about 30 minutes. Add the tamari and simmer for another 10 minutes. Meanwhile, heat the oven to 375°F.

3 Slice the French bread into 2-inch pieces and place them on a greased baking sheet. Sprinkle the grated cheese on top and bake in the oven for about 20 minutes. Serve the soup hot in individual bowls, topped with one or two slices of toasted bread.

• For a vegan version: Omit the grated cheese. Combine 1 teaspoon Italian seasoning with 1 to 2 tablespoons margarine and spread this on the French bread, before toasting it in the oven for 10 to 20 minutes.

Tofu Quiche

Pastry Dough:
1⅔ cups whole wheat flour
¼ cup corn oil
1 tablespoon sesame seeds
About 6 tablespoons chilled sparkling mineral
  water
Filling:
2 tablespoons oil
12 ounces thinly sliced seasonal vegetables
⅔ cup thinly sliced zucchini

9½ ounces firm tofu
¾ cup plus 2 tablespoons water
2 tablespoons tamari
1 to 2 tablespoons nutritional yeast flakes or
  grated vegan cheese (optional)
Pepper to taste
1 red bell pepper, sliced into rings, cored,
  and seeded
Parsley sprigs, to garnish

1 Prepare the dough first. For the best results, make sure all the ingredients are cold. Lightly combine the flour and corn oil, then stir in the sesame seeds. Add enough sparkling water to make a soft dough, but avoid overmixing. Allow to rest (preferably in the refrigerator) for at least 30 minutes. Meanwhile, heat the oven to 400°F.

2 To make the filling, heat the oil in a skillet and sauté the seasonal vegetables for about 5 minutes; set aside. Roll out the dough on a lightly floured surface and use to line a 9-inch tart pan with a removeable bottom. Arrange the sliced zucchini on the dough and the sautéed vegetables on top.

3 Put the tofu, water, tamari, and yeast flakes or cheese, if using, in a food processor or blender and blend until smooth. Season with pepper. Pour the mixture over the vegetables and arrange the red pepper slices on top. Bake in the oven for 40 minutes. Serve hot or cold, garnished with sprigs of parsley.

Pommes de Terre Roti au Romarin

6 to 8 potatoes with skins on
2 to 3 tablespoons olive oil

Salt and pepper
2 to 3 tablespoons crumbled fresh rosemary

1 Heat the oven to 400°F. Scrub the potatoes and slice them thinly. Brush with the oil and place in a roasting pan. Season with salt and pepper and sprinkle the crumbled rosemary over the top.

2 Bake the potatoes in the oven for 80 minutes, turning the slices occasionally.

Petits Pois à la Français

3 cups shelled peas
1 tablespoon butter or margarine, plus extra
   if required

2 or 3 large lettuce leaves
Salt and pepper to taste

1 Place the peas and butter or margarine in a pan. Gently wash the lettuce leaves, taking care to keep them whole. Do not dry them, but gently place them over the peas in the pan with water still clinging to the leaves.

2 Cover the pan and cook over low heat for about 10 minutes, until the peas are tender. Season with salt and pepper and add more butter, if desired.

Prune Mousse

9 ounces dried prunes, pitted
1 cup water
1 tablespoon agar-agar flakes
1 tablespoon honey or date syrup (optional)

2¼ cups creamy yogurt
1 teaspoon lemon juice
¼ cup chopped nuts, to decorate

1 Put the prunes and water in a pan, bring to a boil, and simmer for about 20 minutes, until soft. Transfer to a food processor or blender and blend until smooth.

2 Return the prune purée to the pan, stir in the agar-agar flakes, and simmer for 2 minutes longer; leave to cool slightly.

3 When lukewarm, fold in the honey or date syrup, yogurt, and lemon juice. Pour into individual dishes and chill until set. Decorate with chopped nuts before serving.

• Vegans can substitute Toasted Nut Dream (page 115) for the yogurt.
• Dates or any other dried fruit(s) may be used instead or some, or all, of the prunes.

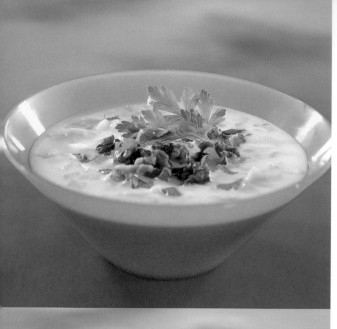

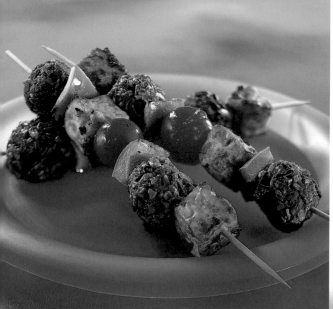

Picnic in the Sun

Chilled Cucumber Soup
Tofu Veggie Kabobs
Cold Sesame Noodles
Salads
Fruit Brochettes
Papaya Zing

Serves 4 to 6

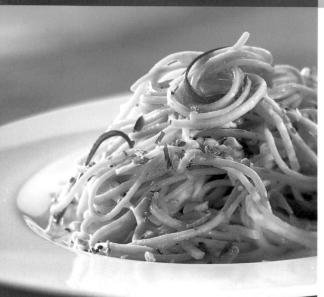

Whether in Australia, the Bahamas, or California, beaches are places of increased concentration of prana—perfect for meditation, asanas, and pranayama, followed by a sattvic feast with friends.

Top left—Chilled Cucumber Soup: Sets the tone for our international picnic.

Center left—Tofu Veggie Kabobs: These can be marinated the day before and barbecued at a nearby lake or seaside, or bake them in the oven and enjoy in your own garden.

Bottom left—Cold Sesame Noodles: These are both smooth and crunchy, a traditional Chinese appetizer.

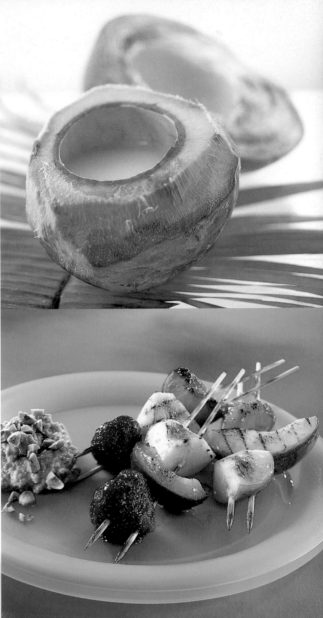

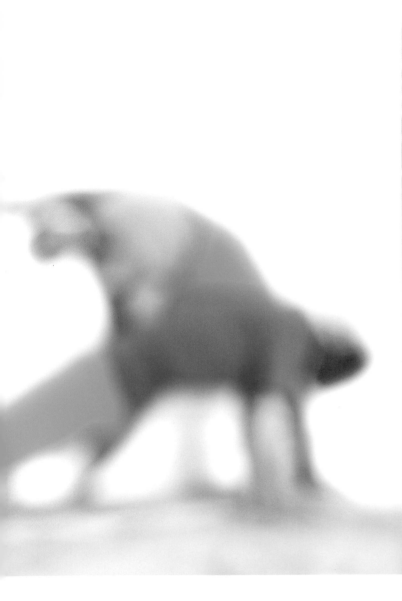

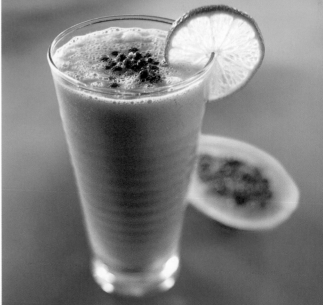

Not pictured—Salads: Coleslaw (page 98) and Potato Salad (page 99) are the perennial picnic favourites, but all salads taste special when eaten outdoors.

Center right—Fruit Brochettes: Very simple to make and any fruits will do.

Bottom right—Papaya Zing: A delicious, refreshing drink to serve as a start or finish to the picnic meal. Papaya, or pawpaw as it is known in the Bahamas, has a sweet-and-slightly-bitter taste and provides a wonderful source of digestive enzymes. Its effect on both the mind and the body is calming and grounding.

Chilled Cucumber Soup

3⅓ cups plain yogurt
½ teaspoon salt
2 tablespoons oil
1 cucumber, peeled and finely chopped
1 to 2 tablespoons lemon juice

½ teaspoon pepper
1 cup iced water
1 cup chopped walnuts
Fresh parsley leaves, to garnish

Combine the yogurt, salt, and oil, stirring until smooth. Add the cucumber, lemon juice, pepper, and iced water. Chill until ready to serve, or add ½ cup chopped ice and serve immediately. Serve topped with a sprinkling of chopped walnuts and garnished with parsley.

Tofu Veggie Kabobs

Tofu cubes:
10 ounces firm tofu (pressed for 30 minutes
   to remove excess moisture)
1 tablespoon olive oil
1 tablespoon tomato paste
½ teaspoon turmeric
Salt and pepper to taste
Eggplant balls:
2 tablespoons margarine
2 sticks of celery, very finely chopped
1 large eggplant, finely diced

1 teaspoon tomato paste
½ teaspoon ground cumin
1 cup pumpkin seeds, toasted and finely
   chopped
1¼ cups fresh whole wheat bread crumbs
To finish:
1 green or red bell pepper (or half of each),
   cut into bite-size pieces
20 to 24 cherry tomatoes
Oil for brushing

1 Cut the tofu into bite-size cubes and place in a dish. Combine the olive oil, tomato paste, turmeric, and salt and pepper to make a marinade. Pour it over the tofu and leave to marinate for about 12 hours.

2 About 1 hour before you want to eat, light the barbecue or heat the oven to 350°F.

3 To make the eggplant balls, melt the margarine in a pan and sauté the celery over medium heat until soft. Add the eggplant and cook to a pulp. Stir in the tomato paste, cumin, pumpkin seeds, and bread crumbs. Season to taste with salt and pepper. Form the eggplant mixture into bite-size balls.

4 Thread the ingredients onto 8 to 12 barbecue skewers, alternating tofu cubes and eggplant balls with pieces of green or red bell pepper and cherry tomatoes.

5 Brush the vegetables with a little oil and cook them on the barbecue, or in the oven, for 15 to 20 minutes, turning the kabobs once or twice during cooking.

Cold Sesame Noodles

12 ounces whole wheat, spinach, or
buckwheat noodles
1½ tablespoons finely grated fresh gingerroot
1½ tablespoons finely grated turnip
1 tablespoon tahini
1½ tablespoons toasted sesame oil
1½ tablespoons chunky peanut butter (optional)

3 tablespoons tamari
4 to 5 tablespoons water
½ to 1 teaspoon mustard powder
1½ tablespoons lemon juice
3 tablespoons maple syrup
¼ red or green bell pepper, cored, seeded, and
cut into slivers, to garnish (optional)

1 Cook the noodles in boiling water until tender but still firm. Drain thoroughly and rinse with cold
water, then chill in the refrigerator for at least 1 hour.

2 Put all the other ingredients in a bowl and whisk together. Leave to stand for a few minutes.
Pour the mixture over the noodles and toss well just before serving. Garnish with slivers of pepper
if you want to add a bit of color.

Fruit Brochettes

1 tablespoon maple syrup or date syrup
1 teaspoon grated lemon zest
2 teaspoons lemon juice
Pinch of freshly grated nutmeg

1¼ to 1½ pounds assorted fruits, in large pieces
(cubed pineapple, quartered nectarines or
peaches, halved apricots, quartered plums,
cubed apples and pears, whole strawberries)
Toasted Nut Dream (page 115) or yogurt, to serve
(optional)

1 Light the barbecue and let it get very hot, or heat the oven to 450°F.

2 Combine the maple or date syrup, lemon zest, lemon juice, and nutmeg in a bowl; set aside.
Thread the cubes of fruit onto barbecue skewers, using two skewers per kabob, and brush with
the syrup mixture.

3 Place on the hot grill for 2 minutes, turning over after 1 minute and brushing with any remaining
syrup. If cooking in the oven, place on a baking sheet and cook for the same time. If you like,
serve with toasted nut dream or yogurt.

Papaya Zing

1 pound ripe papaya, peeled, seeded, and cut
into chunks (retain about 1 tablespoon of the
seeds for decoration)
2 teaspoons fresh lime or lemon juice
Pinch of ground allspice

¾ cup fresh orange juice
2 teaspoons honey (optional)
1 cup buttermilk or soy milk
Lime or lemon slices, to decorate

1 Put all the ingredients, except the decoration, in a food processor or blender and blend until
smooth. Chill in the refrigerator.

2 To serve, pour into individual glasses and decorate with slices of lime or lemon and a few of the
delicious, peppery papaya seeds.

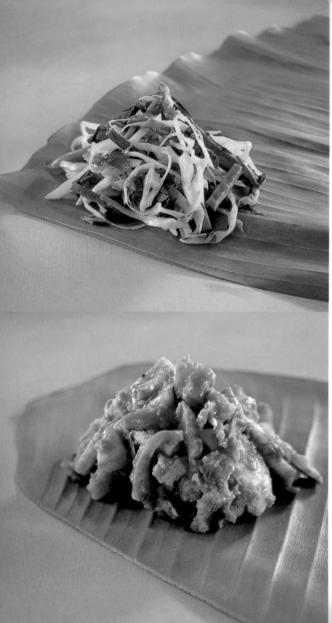

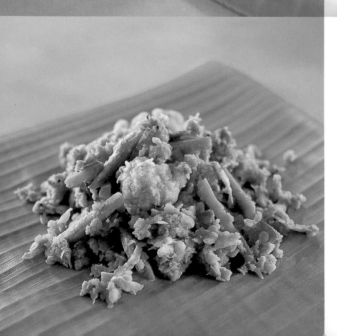

South Indian Bandhara

Plain basmati rice
Sambar
Aviyal
Poduthuval
Pineapple Pachadi
Pappadams
Lemon pickle
Plain yogurt
Paysam
Banana

Serves 4

There is no greater blessing than to be able to give food. This South Indian feast is one that might accompany a birthday party or other "festive" day when we want to share something special with family, friends, and guests.

The main meal is eaten midday and rice is the mainstay. Sambar (pictured bottom left) is poured directly on top of the rice. This delicious high-protein dish has a very liquidy texture and a deliciously earthy, slightly acid taste. Sambar is also served with Dosas or Uppama with Mixed Vegetables (page 28), or a variety of other dishes for a typical South Indian breakfast or light evening supper.

Top left—Poduthuval: Deliciously green.

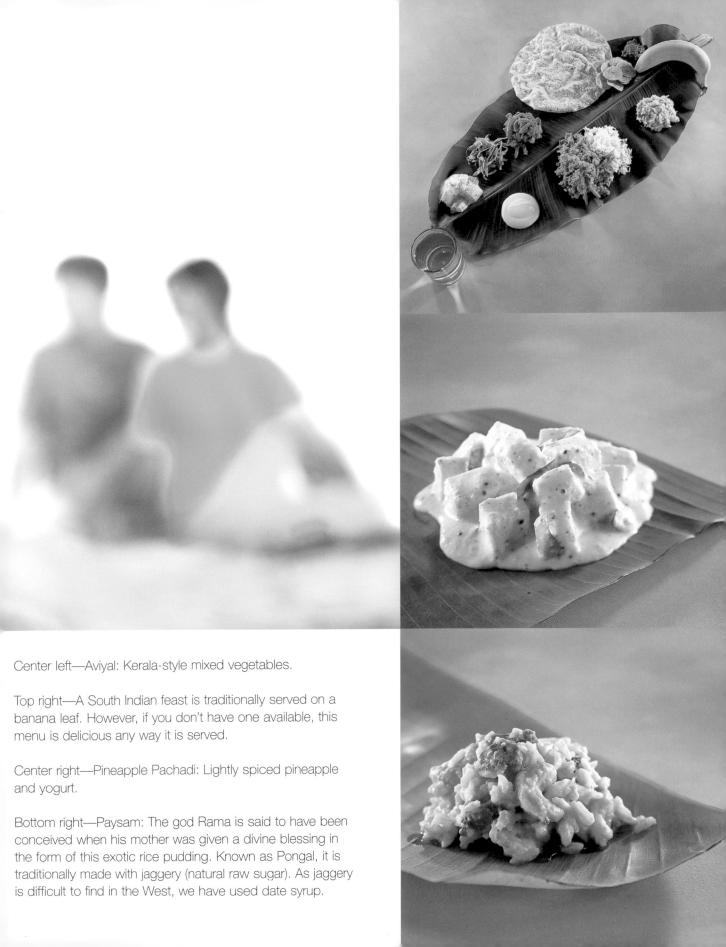

Center left—Aviyal: Kerala-style mixed vegetables.

Top right—A South Indian feast is traditionally served on a banana leaf. However, if you don't have one available, this menu is delicious any way it is served.

Center right—Pineapple Pachadi: Lightly spiced pineapple and yogurt.

Bottom right—Paysam: The god Rama is said to have been conceived when his mother was given a divine blessing in the form of this exotic rice pudding. Known as Pongal, it is traditionally made with jaggery (natural raw sugar). As jaggery is difficult to find in the West, we have used date syrup.

Sambar

1 cup red lentils
1½ quarts water
2 tablespoons ghee or oil
1 teaspoon black mustard seeds
1 teaspoon turmeric
1 teaspoon grated fresh gingerroot
2 green chilies, seeded and finely chopped
4 teaspoons sambar powder, or 2 teaspoons
    ground cumin, 2 teaspoons ground coriander,
    and ½ teaspoon cayenne pepper

2 tablespoons grated fresh coconut
½ cup cauliflower flowerets
½ cup green beans cut into 1-inch pieces
½ cup cubed eggplant
½ cup carrots cut into batons
½ cup cored, seeded, and chopped green
    bell pepper
½ cup chopped tomatoes
2 teaspoons salt
2 tablespoons lemon juice

1 Place the lentils in a large pan with the water and bring to a boil. Half cover and simmer for 20 to 30 minutes, until the lentils are soft; set the lentils aside in the water they have been cooked in.

2 Heat the ghee or oil in a large skillet. Add the mustard seeds and cook over high heat until they "pop." Add the rest of the spices, then the coconut and cook for 5 minutes, stirring.

3 Add the vegetables and sauté for about 5 minutes. Add to the cooked lentils along with the salt and simmer for 5 to 10 minutes, until the vegetables are soft. Add the lemon juice, stir well, and serve hot.

• Substitute toor dal or pigeon peas (also called Congo peas) for the red lentils.

Aviyal

1¼ pounds mixed vegetables (potatoes,
    plantains, Indian drumsticks (page 156), carrots,
    green bell peppers), cut into julienne strips
1 cup water
½ teaspoon salt
1 teaspoon tamarind concentrate

2 tablespoons unsweetened dried coconut
2 green chilies, seeded
½ teaspoon cumin seeds
1 teaspoon coconut oil
3 or 4 curry leaves (page 156), shredded

1 Place the mixed vegetables in a pan with the water and bring to a boil. Cover and simmer for 10 minutes. Remove from the heat, drain off the water, and reserve it.

2 Place the salt, tamarind concentrate, shredded coconut, green chilies, and cumin seeds in a food processor or blender with the reserved vegetable cooking water. Blend finely, then pour this mixture over the vegetables and stir well to coat them. Cover and cook over low heat for 10 minutes. Remove from the heat and add the coconut oil and curry leaves. Serve hot (keep covered if not serving immediately). To eat the drumstick julienne, suck the flesh off the skin and discard the skin.

Poduthuval

1 tablespoon oil
½ teaspoon mustard seeds
½ teaspoon urid dal or white lentils
1 red chili, broken in half
½ teaspoon turmeric

13 to 14 ounces mixed green vegetables
(green beans, Chinese long beans, cabbage,
spinach), finely shredded
½ teaspoon salt
4 tablespoons water

1 Heat the oil in a pan, add the mustard seeds, urid dal or lentils, and chili and cook over high heat until the mustard seeds "pop" and the dal is a golden brown.

2 Add the turmeric, mixed vegetables, salt, and water. Cover and cook over medium heat for 5 to 6 minutes, until the vegetables are tender. Remove from the heat, discard the chili halves, and keep the pan covered until ready to serve the vegetables.

Pineapple Pachadi

2 tablespoons unsweetened dried coconut
1 green chili, seeded and chopped
Pinch of mustard seeds
½ pineapple, peeled, cored, and cut into small
chunks

½ cup plain yogurt
½ teaspoon ghee
½ teaspoon black mustard seeds
1 or 2 curry leaves, shredded
¼ teaspoon salt

1 Place the coconut, chili, and pinch of mustard seeds in a blender and grind finely. Mix this powder with the pineapple chunks and yogurt.

2 Heat the ghee in a small skillet. Add the black mustard seeds and roast them until they "pop." Pour the seeds over the pineapple mixture. Stir in the curry leaves and salt.

Paysam

4½ cups milk or soy milk
3 cardamom pods
⅓ cup basmati rice, rinsed

2 tablespoons cashew nuts
3 tablespoons raisins
⅓ cup date syrup or honey

1 Bring the milk almost to the boil in a pan, reduce the heat to low, and simmer it for 15 to 20 minutes, stirring frequently.

2 Remove the seeds from the cardamom pods, discarding the husks. Crush the seeds slightly and add to the milk. Add the rice, cashew nuts, and raisins. Cover the pan and continue to cook over low heat for about 20 to 30 minutes, until the rice is soft. Remove from the heat, stir in the date syrup or honey and serve.

• Add a pinch of ground saffron with the rice, if desired. Vermicelli may be used instead of basmati rice.

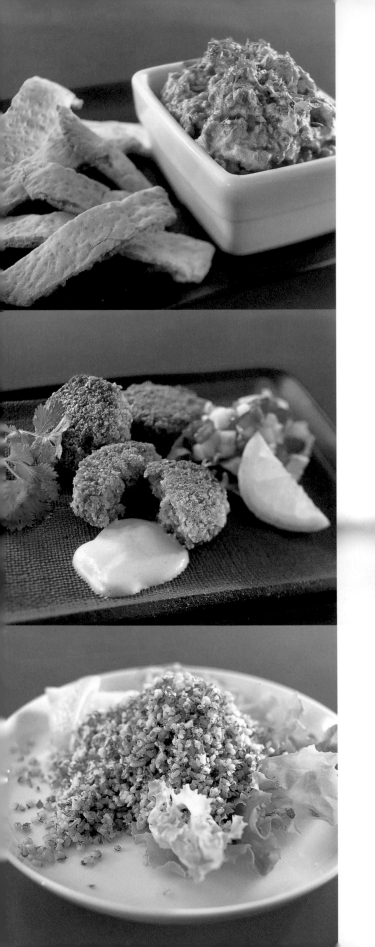

Middle Eastern Feast

Baba Ganoush with pita bread
Falafel with Tahini Sauce
Tabbouleh
Cucumber, Dill, and Yogurt Salad
Fragrant Fruit Salad

Serves 4 to 6

Middle Eastern meals tend to be salad orientated. These recipes were contributed by the very active Sivananda Yoga Centre in Tel Aviv and our strong Lebanese contingent in Montreal. They may be augmented by a variety of other salads and dishes, such as Mediterranean Salad (page 98).

Top left—Baba Ganoush: A cool eggplant dish with a smoky, exotic flavor. It is served with warm pita bread.

Center left—Falafel with Tahini Sauce: The perennial favorite sandwich filling of the Middle East. Falafel is lovely served with either tahini or yogurt sauce.

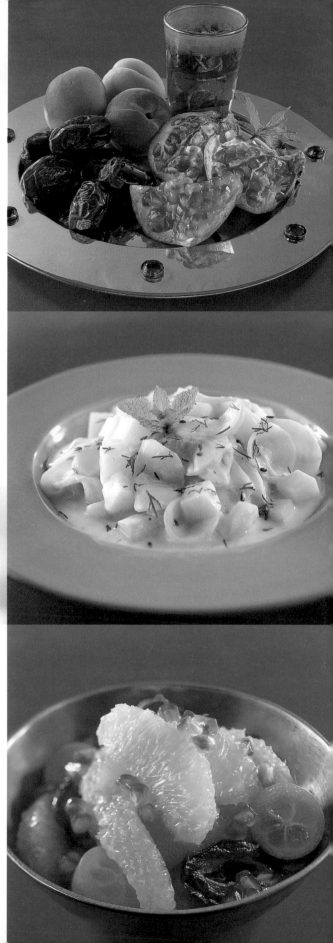

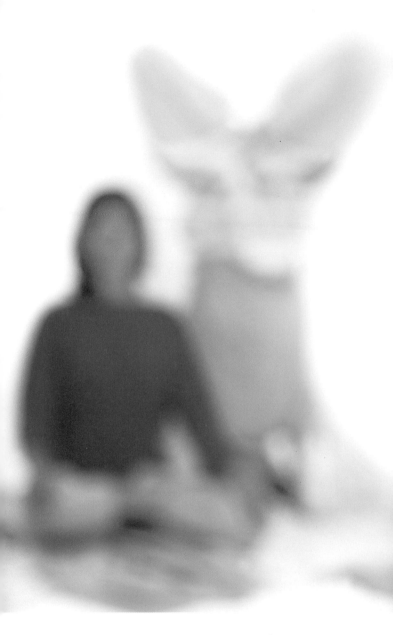

Bottom left—Tabbouleh: A popular grain salad made with lots of chopped fresh mint and parsley. It is delightful on its own for a light summer supper or combined with other dishes.

Center right—Cucumber, Dill, and Yogurt Salad: Rejuvenates the palate.

Bottom right—Fragrant Fruit Salad: A deliciously refreshing citrus salad of oranges, grapefruit, kumquats, and dates, delicately flavored with orange-flower water.

Baba Ganoush

1 large eggplant
2 tablespoons tahini
2 tablespoons olive oil
Juice of 1 lemon
Salt and pepper to taste

Paprika
2 to 3 sprigs of mint or parsley, coarsely chopped
Pita bread, to serve (optional)

1 Heat the oven to 375°F. Prick the eggplant to prevent the skin bursting, then place it in a baking dish and bake in the oven for 45 to 60 minutes, or until the flesh inside is very soft.

2 Leave the eggplant to cool, then peel it. Mash the flesh, leaving it in a strainer for a few minutes to drain off the excess juice. When drained, transfer it to a bowl. Beat the tahini, olive oil, and lemon juice together and stir it into the eggplant purée, mixing thoroughly. Season with salt and pepper.

3 Sprinkle a little paprika over the top and garnish with chopped mint or parsley. If serving as a dip, serve with pita bread.

• Omit the tahini and use double the quantity of olive oil (or vice versa).
• Use a different vegetable as a base, such as butternut squash, but this is not traditionally Middle Eastern.

Falafel with Tahini Sauce

Generous 1 cup chick-peas, soaked
Generous 1 cup dried fava beans, soaked
8 tablespoons finely chopped fresh parsley
8 tablespoons finely chopped fresh cilantro
8 tablespoons finely chopped fresh mint
½ teaspoon pepper
1 teaspoon allspice
1 teaspoon salt
1 teaspoon baking powder
Oil for frying

Tahini sauce:
1 cup tahini
1 cup water
Juice of 1 lemon
1 teaspoon salt
To serve and garnish:
Shredded lettuce
Chopped tomatoes and cucumber
Lemon wedges
Cilantro sprigs

1 To make the falafel, drain the chick-peas and beans. Put them in a food processor with the herbs, pepper, allspice, and salt and blend until they are the consistency of fine bulgur wheat. Add the baking powder and leave to rest for at least 1 hour.

2 Meanwhile, to make the sauce, combine all the ingredients in a bowl.

3 Heat the oil in a skillet. Form small balls of chick-pea mixture and flatten them slightly between the palms of the hands. Fry them, in batches, in the hot oil for 3 minutes, or until golden brown. Drain on paper towels.

4 Serve the falafel with shredded lettuce, chopped tomatoes, and cucumber, garnished with lemon wedges and cilantro sprigs, and accompanied by the tahini sauce.

Tabbouleh

1 cup bulgur wheat
½ cup boiling water
2 cups finely chopped fresh parsley
2 cups finely chopped fresh mint
Juice of 2 lemons

⅔ cup olive oil
Sea salt and pepper to taste
1 teaspoon ground cinnamon
Lettuce leaves, to serve
Lemon wedges, to garnish

1 Place the bulgur wheat in a large mixing bowl and pour the boiling water over it. Cover tightly and leave for 30 to 40 minutes, until the water is absorbed and the grains are soft and fluffy.

2 Mix in all the remaining ingredients, except the lettuce leaves and lemon wedges. Serve the salad on a bed of lettuce leaves, garnished with lemon wedges.

• Omit the cinnamon and add a peeled and finely chopped cucumber.

Cucumber, Dill, and Yogurt Salad

1 teaspoon cumin seeds
2 tablespoons lemon juice
1 tablespoon fresh dill or 1 teaspoon dried
   dillweed
2¼ cups plain yogurt

Pinch of cayenne pepper
½ teaspoon salt
3 cups peeled and thinly sliced cucumber
2 potatoes, cooked and diced (optional)
Fresh mint leaves, to garnish

1 Toast the cumin seeds in a hot, dry skillet over high heat until the aroma starts to appear. Remove from the heat and crush the seeds slightly with a rolling pin.

2 Mix the seeds with the lemon juice, dill, yogurt, cayenne, and salt in a large bowl. Stir in the cucumber slices and diced potatoes, if using. Serve garnished with mint leaves.

• **Yogurt Sauce:** Omit the cooked potatoes and the cucumber.
• **Cucumber Raita:** Omit the mint and dill and add 1 bunch of cilantro leaves. Serve with Indian meals.

Fragrant Fruit Salad

2 oranges
½ teaspoon orange-flower water
1 to 2 tablespoons honey or date syrup (optional)
1 pink grapefruit

8 kumquats, halved, or 16 cherries
1 cup fresh dates or figs, halved and
   cut lengthwise
Pomegranate seeds

1 Squeeze the juice from one orange and combine it with the orange-flower water and honey or date syrup, if using, to make a syrup. Remove all skin and pith from the other orange and the grapefruit, dividing them into segments.

2 Arrange the fruits in a bowl and pour the syrup over them. Sprinkle with pomegranate seeds and chill before serving.

• If fresh figs or dates are unavailable, use dried, and soak in cold water for 30 minutes.

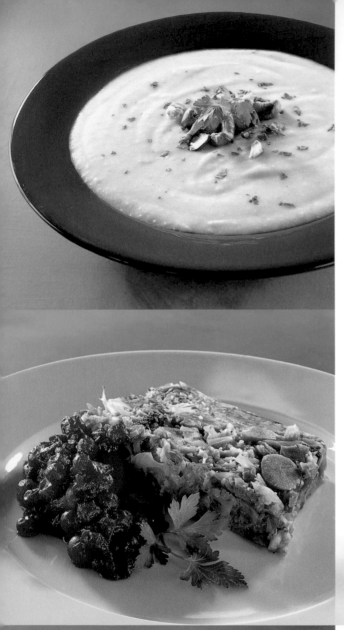

Winter Festival

Celery Root and Cashew Soup
Green salad with Seeded Yogurt Dressing
Chestnut Roast with Rich Brown Gravy and
Cranberry Sauce
Steamed Brussels sprouts and/or broccoli
Sweet Potato with Pineapple
Carrot and Parsnip Julienne
Plum Pudding
Holiday Punch
Rich Tofu Fruit Cake

Serves 6 to 8

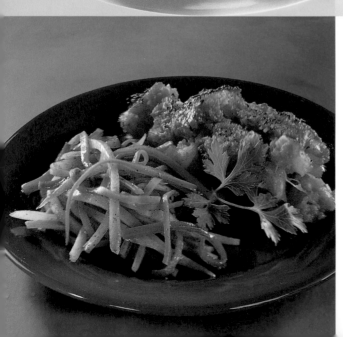

Throughout the world there are times of particular joy. The Sivananda Yoga Center in New York has perfected the vegetarian adaptations of the traditional Thanksgiving and Christmas meal at their annual feasts.

Top left—Celery Root and Cashew Soup (page 39) is followed by a green salad topped with Seeded Yogurt Dressing (pictured on page 121).

Center left—Chestnut Roast with its chunky, rich texture is a vegan's delight. Here it is shown with Cranberry Sauce (page 125). It is also served with Rich Brown Gravy (page 122).

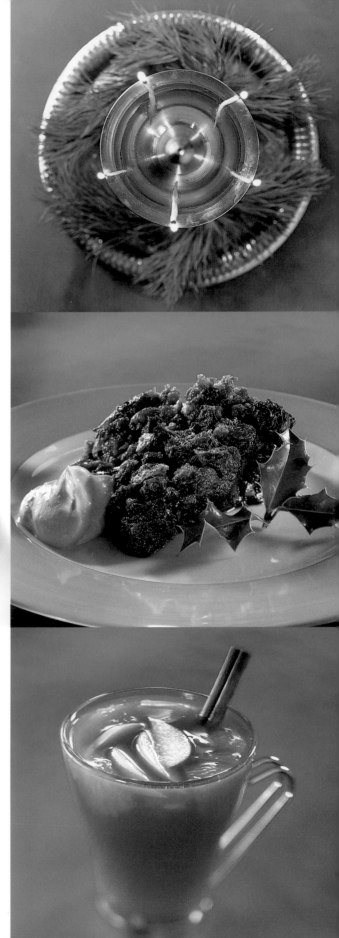

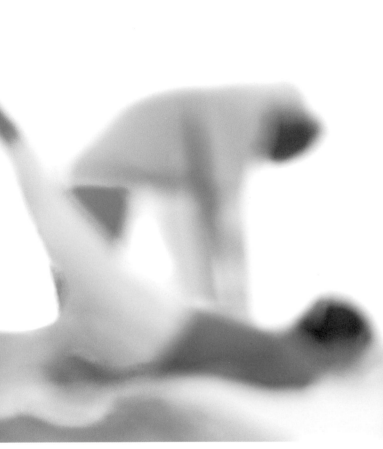

Bottom left—Sweet Potato with Pineapple: Not a dessert, but a traditional part of American Thanksgiving meals, pictured here with Carrot and Parsnip Julienne. Steamed Brussels sprouts and/or broccoli (not pictured) are also served.

Center right—Plum Pudding: A zesty, healthy version of a traditional, old-fashioned recipe, much richer in fruit and nuts than anything you can buy.

Bottom right—Holiday Punch: A deliciously warming drink to serve before the meal as a toast—or later with Rich Tofu Fruitcake (page 114).

Chestnut Roast

1 pound fresh chestnuts
2 cups mixed nuts (unsalted almonds
  and brazil nuts are best)
1 cup millet
2¾ cups water
2 tablespoons oil
2 carrots, grated
½ cabbage, finely sliced
2 sticks of celery, chopped
9 ounces broccoli, the top broken into flowerets
  and the stems chopped

3 tablespoons tomato paste
2 tablespoons tamari
¼ teaspoon pepper
1 tablespoon dried Italian seasoning
Slivered almonds, pumpkin seeds, and parsley
  sprigs, to garnish
Rich Brown Gravy (page 122) and Cranberry Sauce
  (page 125), to serve

1 Heat the oven to 375°F. To peel the chestnuts, make a small slit in the pointed end. Place them in a pan, cover with boiling water, and leave for 5 minutes. Remove them from the water, one at a time, and peel off the thick outer skin and thin inner skin while warm. Cook the peeled chestnuts in boiling water for about 30 minutes, until soft; set aside, reserving the water for stock.

2 Meanwhile, spread out the mixed nuts on a baking sheet and toast in the oven for about 10 minutes, until lightly brown, stirring from time to time. Coarsely chop the nuts; set aside. Cook the millet in the water (page 46); set aside.

3 Heat the oil in a pan and add the carrots, cabbage, and celery. Cover and cook over medium heat for a few minutes, then add the broccoli and cook for 1 to 2 minutes. Add the tomato paste, tamari, pepper, Italian seasoning, chestnuts, mixed nuts, and cooked millet. Stir in enough reserved stock to bind everything together.

4 Transfer the mixture to a greased 9- x 5-inch bread pan and bake in the oven for about 45 minutes. Garnish with flaked almonds, pumpkin seeds and parsley sprigs and serve with gravy and cranberry sauce.

Sweet Potatoes with Pineapple

5 large sweet potatoes, total weight about
  3¼ pounds
2 tablespoons butter or margarine
1 very ripe fresh pineapple, about 2¼ pounds

⅔ cup orange juice
1 teaspoon ground cardamom
½ teaspoon salt

1 Heat the oven to 375°F. Scrub the sweet potatoes and bake them for 1 to 1½ hours, until soft. (These may be put in the oven while it is hot for the chestnut roast.)

2 Remove the sweet potatoes from the oven and reduce the temperature to 275°F. Leave the potatoes until cool enough to handle, then peel and mash them with the butter or margarine. Peel and core the pineapple, using a sharp knife. Cut into small pieces. Combine the mashed potatoes, pineapple, and other ingredients. Transfer to a baking dish and bake for about 40 minutes. Serve hot.

Carrot and Parsnip Julienne

3 cups carrots cut into julienne
3 cups parsnips cut into julienne
6 tablespoons orange juice
6 tablespoons water
2 tablespoons butter or oil
1 tablespoon lemon juice

¼ teaspoon ground ginger
1 teaspoon freshly grated nutmeg
Pinch of salt
Pepper
2 tablespoons maple syrup
Parsley sprigs, to garnish

Place all the ingredients, except the maple syrup and garnish, in a pan and simmer over low heat for 15 minutes. Leave on a low heat and add the maple syrup, stirring gently until the vegetables are glazed. Serve hot, garnished with parsley.

Plum Pudding

1 cup chopped dates
1⅓ cup raisins
1⅓ cup currants
1⅓ cup golden raisins
1 cup chopped prunes
1 cup mixed peel
Generous 1 cup Barbados sugar (or use extra dates and barley malt syrup instead)
¼ teaspoon freshly grated nutmeg

½ teaspoon apple-pie spice
3 cups fresh whole wheat bread crumbs
½ cup chopped almonds
8 ounces vegetable suet
Scant ½ cup whole wheat flour
1 cup plus 3 tablespoons orange juice, plus extra if necessary
Tofu Whipped Dream or Toasted Nut Dream (page 115), to serve (optional)

1 Wash the dried fruit and place it in a large mixing bowl. Stir in all the dry ingredients and then the orange juice. Cover and leave to stand overnight.

2 The next day, stir the batter—the consistency should be soft and firm, not runny. Add more orange juice if necessary. Press the mixture into a greased 5-cup English-style pudding basin or other heatproof bowl. Cover the top with two layers of waxed paper or a pudding cloth and secure with string.

3 Stand the pudding basin in a large pan with 3 to 4 inches of boiling water in the bottom. Cover the pan tightly and steam the pudding over low heat for about 2 hours, checking from time to time and adding more water to prevent it from boiling dry. Turn out the pudding and serve with tofu whipped dream or toasted nut dream, if desired.

Holiday Punch

4½ cups cranberry juice
4½ cups apple juice
5 or 6 strips of lemon peel
1- to 2-inch piece of fresh gingerroot, peeled and coarsely chopped
2 large cinnamon sticks, broken into pieces

10 to 12 whole cloves
2¼ cups freshly squeezed orange juice
2 crisp eating apples, sliced
2 oranges or satsumas, divided into segments or coarsely chopped
Honey to taste (optional)

Combine the cranberry and apple juices with the lemon peel and spices in a heavy pan. Bring them almost to a boil, then lower the heat and simmer for 10 to 15 minutes. Stir in the orange juice and fruit and add a little honey, if desired. Serve immediately.

FASTING

"Verily Yoga is not possible for the person
who eats too much, nor for the one who does
not eat at all, nor for the one who sleeps too
much, nor the person who is always awake."

Bhagavad Gita, VI. 16

Fasting is one of Nature's greatest healing agents, often restoring health when everything else has failed. It gives a rest to the entire system, giving the body the time to cleanse itself thoroughly, often eliminating impurities that have accumulated for years.

If you constantly overwork the body and mind, without getting proper rest, your system will eventually break down. The digestive system also needs its rest; fasting is a vacation from food.

Fasting is really a rapid curing agent for numerous ailments. It permits the entire digestive system to rest while ridding the body of many toxins. It cleanses the body and makes it much more energetic. Even a one-day fast gives a respite. The body feels lighter. During a fast, the bodily energy that is usually directed toward digestion is available for the repair and healing of the body.

"Yogis advocate occasional fasts, especially during sickness, in order to rest the stomach. The recuperative energy may thereby be directed toward the casting out of the toxins and poisonous matter that have been causing trouble. Nature's precaution of fasting to restore health is to be noted even in animals. They stop eating while they are sick, and lie around until they are normal again, when they return to their food."

Swami Vishnu-devananda,
The Complete Illustrated Book of Yoga

"Both fasting and feasting are blessings to human beings. The feast gives you an immediate blessing, which vanishes in a few hours, inducing a craving for more, whereas a fast gives you a different kind of happiness, more lasting than a feast."

Swami Sivananda,
Health and Diet, Science of Yoga, Volume 7

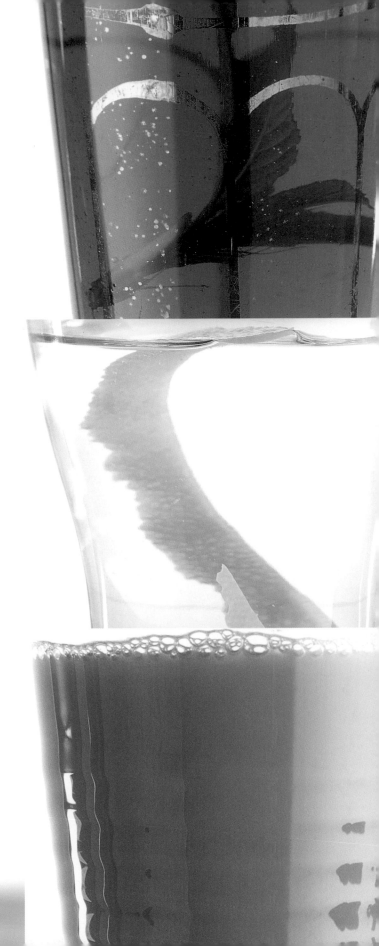

Never confuse fasting with starvation. Fasting is an austerity; it is undertaken voluntarily for a specific purpose, usually to cleanse the system, regain health, or for spiritual clarity. Beautiful for its simplicity, fasting strengthens the mind and the willpower. Just as we can strengthen our muscles by giving them progressively more work to do, so we can also strengthen the mind by giving it increasingly difficult tasks to perform. Fasting will help in the development of concentration and mental strength.

Think of the time and energy spent in the preparation and consumption of food. During a fast, this time is available for other pursuits. When the body and mind are not taken over three times a day by the vibration of food, they are left free to focus on spiritual matters. Fasting assists in the attainment of clear insight. All the religions of the world recommend fasting, often with vigil, as a means of strengthening prayer. We are reminded of how Christ went into the desert to fast and pray for 40 days.

Many yogis fast twice a month on "Ekadasi" days, the eleventh day of each of the lunar fortnights. Considered especially auspicious for the practices of fasting and meditation, the observance of Ekadasi is based on the effects of the Moon on body and mind.

We are aware of the Moon's influence on the tides. As our bodies are 75 percent water, its effects may be observed in them as well. Without an awareness of this influence, many aspects of our lives seem beyond our control. We are dragged along by the forces of Nature. But a person who understands the effect, and uses it to empower his/her life, may be said to be practicing yoga. Even more than the body, the mind is forcefully affected as the Moon waxes and wanes. The influence is so powerful the Moon is viewed as the presiding deity of the mind.

For the purpose of meditation, there is a great advantage in keeping the body light and the stomach free. This tapas (austerity) helps in gaining control of the mind and strengthening the willpower. Fasting is supposed to cause a buoyant feeling. People who cannot observe a total fast may take light foods on Ekadasi days, but avoid grains as they are more difficult to digest than fruit or vegetables.

CAUTION

Although fasting is an excellent remedy, it should not be expected to accomplish the impossible. It cannot cure deficiency diseases that result from insufficient nourishment or congenital defects. Do not fast if you are pregnant, if you suffer from anemia or diabetes, or if you have had an eating disorder. Consult your doctor if you are in doubt.

How to Fast

A total fast means abstinence from all food, in either liquid or solid form. Water is not a food; it does not stimulate the appetite and it does not need to be digested. It is important to drink plenty of water during a fast as it helps to cleanse the body and flush the toxins out of your system.

When you fast do not entertain thoughts of food. You will not derive the full benefits of fasting if your mind always dwells on food. Fasting is a golden opportunity to turn your thoughts toward God. Entertain sublime, divine thoughts.

Keep yourself busy with peaceful activities during the fast. The practice of asanas and pranayama will help you in the elimination of toxins. You will be surprised to find how much more limber your body becomes when it is not taking in food.

Rest and relax as much as possible. Try to be quiet and to spend time by yourself whenever you can.

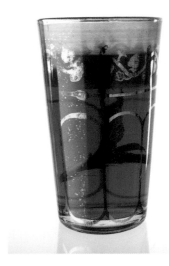

Hot peppermint tea is good for helping to banish a headache or nausea when fasting.

Possible Side Effects

• The tongue may feel furry while fasting. Many yogis use tongue cleaners to remove the toxins that exit the body via the tongue. Brushing your teeth or rinsing your mouth frequently also helps.

• Fasting is also an excellent time to learn, and to practice, kriyas. These are yogic cleansing techniques; they are quite easy to do, but are best learned from a teacher.

• Sometimes, especially when you are new to fasting, you may experience some side effects. If you have a headache or nausea, drink some hot peppermint tea. Do not drink regular tea or coffee.

• The stomach will cease to feel hungry after the third day of the fast. Peristaltic action will slow down and/or stop in the small intestine.

• You may experience some constipation during a fast. The daily use of an enema is recommended during the period of the fast, and for a day or two afterward, if it is necessary.

• You may feel cold, because the body is not taking in the usual calories (heat units). The process of digestion itself warms the body, as does activity and movement. Many people feel chilled when they are fasting and the body is still. Be careful to keep yourself warm.

• You may feel very sensitive or hyperemotional, as the fast helps to cleanse the emotional as well as physical impurities. Be aware of this and do not allow swings of emotion to affect you.

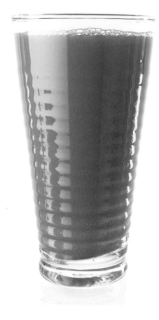

Some people prefer to fast on raw vegetable and/or fruit juices, which are a good way of detoxifying the body.

Juice Fast

Some people prefer to fast on raw vegetable juices and/or fruit juices. Although not technically a fast, juicing is an excellent way to detoxify the body, gain willpower, and strengthen the mind.

There are advantages and disadvantages to juice fasting. Juices insulate you a bit against the stresses and strains of the outside world; they nourish the body and provide stamina. Carrot juice, the most popular for a fast, is an energy drink. It can be drunk alone or mixed with other vegetable juices for a tasty pick-me-up (for example, see Ginger Carrot Juice on page 22). However, one disadvantage is that juices stimulate digestion, so you feel more hungry on a juice fast. Also, as juices speed up detoxification, more people experience headaches and other side effects when doing a juice fast. However, even for the novice, a one-day-a-week juice fast is excellent.

"Raw, freshly made vegetable and fruit juices are very good for those who suffer from chronic ailments. Do not think that raw vegetable juices are like drugs to cure ailments. They are rather the most vital rebuilding and regenerating foods that the body can use for construction. The raw fruits and vegetables are the storehouses of nature's energy to nourish the starved cells of the body. When one intends to fast for a week or two on only freshly made juice, one can drink several pints of juice a day. At times one can feel discomfort from fasting on raw juices, usually because of the stirring up of poisons accumulated in the system, which nature is anxious to eliminate, but energy and vigor return when the toxin is eliminated."

Swami Vishnu-devananda, The Complete Illustrated Book of Yoga

When and How Long to Fast

• If you are new to fasting, it is best to begin with a short fast. If you are under age, discuss with your parents first.

• Fasting on a regular basis helps to keep the body and mind healthy.

• Even beginners may safely fast for 1 to 3 days without the guidance of an expert. Pick a time when you can be quiet, perhaps at the weekend. You may choose to be on your own, or with a group who are also fasting and will reinforce your resolve.

• One day of fasting each week maintains good health and mental resolve.

• Weekend fasts are recommended several times per year, especially at the times when the seasons are changing.

• Long fasts of a week or more give great spiritual strength. After the third day, you will probably find your hunger disappears; fast until your normal hunger returns.

A Weekend Fast

Many Sivananda Yoga centers run Fasting Weekends. We advise students to have a light lunch on Friday and no evening meal. On Saturday and Sunday, they take only water and herb teas. We have an official "break-fast" on Sunday evening after satsang. This is a communal meal, always enjoyed by all. Most people agree they have never tasted anything better than the stewed apples served at that meal. They are then advised to follow a regime of reintroducing foods in their diet, and invited back for a "reunion" meal on Friday, their first day back on a full, hopefully healthy, diet.

When and How to Break the Fast

Many people believe that the correct breaking of the fast is more important, and more difficult, than the actual fast itself. The mind may develop abnormal cravings for foods. Be careful to resist these impulses. It is best to begin eating slowly. Do not take heavy food all of a sudden. Nature takes her own time and course to renovate and invigorate the body.

Eating juicy raw or stewed fresh fruit is a very good way to break the fast.

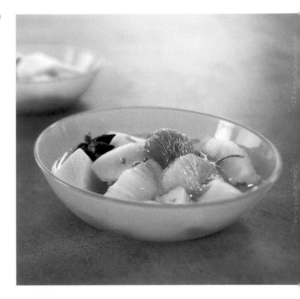

Day 1: Eat only fresh, peeled fruits, either raw or stewed. Juicy fruits, like apples or grapes, are easy to digest and will help to gently restart the peristaltic action of the digestive system. Do not take starchy fruits, such as bananas, or oily fruits like coconuts. Chew your food very slowly and thoroughly. You will experience an absolute calmness and a feeling of happiness that can never be expressed.

Day 2: Add a meal of raw vegetable salad. This will act as a broom to sweep out the toxins that have accumulated in the intestines.

Day 3: In addition to the fruits and raw vegetables, include lightly steamed vegetables in your diet. Do not add salt or any seasonings to the food.

Day 4: Add grains to your diet.

Day 5: You may return to a fully balanced diet, but try to refrain from returning to unhealthy habits such as coffee, tea, alcohol, and meat.

If the fast is not broken properly and the stomach is overloaded by eating too much and too heavy foods, you may get bloated. To get rid of this condition, fast again. Take hot baths and one or more enemas daily. When the swelling disappears, break the fast; this time do it slowly and carefully.

Glossary

Agar-agar: (also known as agar or kanten): A seaweed setting agent or "gel," available in strands, blocks, or powder. Agar is sold in most health-food stores and Asian markets.

Ahimsa: The basic yogic principle of non-violence toward and reverence for all life.

Ake miso: Red miso made from soybeans mixed with barley. Has a rich, savory flavor.

Annamaya kosha: The physical body or "food" sheath. According to yogic philosophy, each person also has an astral (or subtle) body and a causal body (where the karma is stored).

Arame: A mild-flavored seaweed (or sea vegetable) that does not need to be cooked before eating. You can soak it in water to use in salads, or add to cooked vegetable or grain dishes for added flavor and nutritional value. Arame is available from health-food stores and Asian markets.

Arrowroot: A flavorless, white powdered root used as a thickener in sauces and desserts. High in calcium. Mix arrowroot with a little cold water before adding to hot mixtures. It is available in health-food stores, Asian markets, and supermarkets.

Asana: Yoga physical exercise, whose purpose is to improve control over the mind and promote good health. In Sanskrit, the ancient Indian language, the word means posture or position.

Ashram: A quiet place or monastery where one practices and studies yoga.

Ayurveda: A traditional Indian medical system, based on a principle of focusing on and balancing the subtle energies.

Barley malt syrup: Made from sprouted barley grain, this is a natural sweetener with about 80 percent of the sweetness of honey. It is sold in most health-food stores. Other common grain "malt" sweeteners come from rice and corn.

Besan: Chick-pea flour; often used to add a nutty, pleasant taste to curries, fritters, and desserts. Look for it in health-food stores or Asian food stores.

Bhagavad Gita: The best known of all yogic scriptures.

Carob: Chocolate-like powder from the pulp of the dried carob bean. It is rich in natural sugar, calcium, and other minerals.

Curry leaves: The green leaves of the curry plant, sold by herbal mail-order suppliers and in Asian food stores. There is not a good substitute; if unavailable, omit.

Dal: The Indian term for dried legumes; also refers to the dish made using the legumes.

Drumsticks: Unripe seed pods of a small tree native to India. These resemble long, ridged green beans. Best boiled and then the flesh is sucked or scraped off the fiber. Sold in Indian food stores.

Dulse: Seaweed, exceptionally high in iodine and manganese; traditionally used in soups and as a condiment.

Ekadasi: The eleventh day of each lunar fortnight. Many yogis consider these to be auspicious days for fasting.

Garam masala: An aromatic blend of spices, to be used in moderation in Indian cooking. Curry powder can be used instead, but the flavor will be different.

Ghee: Indian cooking fat, like clarified butter. The butter is heated and the solids removed, leaving only the pure butter oil. Ghee is available in Indian food stores and some delicatessens.

Gomasio: Sesame salt, a condiment high in calcium, iron, and vitamin A and B vitamins. Can replace salt as a flavoring.

Gunas: The three qualities of Nature: Sattva, Rajas, and Tamas. According to yogic philosophy, everything is made up of the gunas in different proportions.

Hatcho: Strongly flavored, dark brown soybean miso.

Hijiki: Black seaweed with a strong taste; excellent source of calcium, iron, and iodine.

Jaggery: The dark brown, dehydrated juice of the sugar cane; full of minerals. Available in Indian food stores.

Karma: The literal translation of this Sanskrit word is "action," which is understood to also include the reaction.

Kombu: A member of the kelp family of seaweeds, yellow-brown in color. It greatly increases the nutritional value of any dish it is added to.

Kome: A variety of white miso made with rice.

Kriyas: Yogic cleansing exercises. Many people find it beneficial to practice kriyas while fasting.

Kuzu: (or kudzo): Powdered tuber often used as a thickener in gravies and stews. Kuzu is soothing to the digestive system.

Lacto-vegetarians: People who refrain from eating meat, fish, and eggs, but do include dairy products in their diet. The yogic diet is a lacto-vegetarian one.

Lecithin: A cell builder, usually extracted from soybeans, which also helps to break down the cholesterol in food. It is a natural binding agent and can be used in baking and in salad dressings.

Mantra: Sanskrit syllables, words, or phrases, repeated while meditating to bring the person to a higher state of consciousness.

Miso: A cultured paste, usually made from soybeans. High in protein, and a natural source of vitamin B12, miso is tasty and very salty. It may be enriched with grains, such as wheat, barley, or rice. It can be diluted with hot water for a quick cup of soup, or used as a flavoring in a variety of dishes. Available as a very thick paste which can be stored in the refrigerator for months. Never boil miso because that destroys the vitamin content.

Molasses: The nutritive part of the sugar cane after the refined white sugar has been removed. This is a good sweetener for baking. Available in all health-food stores and supermarkets. Make sure you buy the unsulfured type. Blackstrap molasses is exceptionally high in iron, and helps to prevent anemia.

Mugi: Red miso made with barley.

Nori: Dark-jade colored seaweed with very high protein content and rich in vitamins A and B1. Nori comes in sheets and can be used as it is, or toasted over a low flame and crumbled into soups, stews, and salads, or eaten plain.

Om: The OM symbol (see page 8) is the yogic's sacred symbol. The syllable OM is the original mantra, the root of all sounds and letters, and thus of all language and thought. To chant the OM mantra, the sound "O" is started deep within the body and then slowly brought upward to join the sound "M" which then resonates through the head.

Pappadams: Thin, round waferlike discs, usually made from lentil or other flours. They are usually fried or roasted over an open fire, and served as a crispy accompaniment to Indian meals. Available from Indian food stores and some supermarkets.

Phyllo pastry: Fine, flaky pastry. The dough is sold in sheets and used extensively in Eastern European and Middle Eastern cooking.

Prana: The vital energy or life force.

Pranayama: Yogic breathing exercises to control the prana.

Prasad: Blessed food, usually eaten at the end of each satsang.

Rajas (rajasic): One of the three gunas; this is the quality of over-activity and passion. Rajasic food is avoided on the yogic diet.

Sadhana: Spiritual practice.

Sadhus: People whose main focus in life is spiritual practice.

Salted black beans: Small black soybeans preserved in salt. Sold in Chinese food stores. The beans are used mainly for seasoning.

Satsang: Literal meaning is "company of the wise," but it is often used to refer to group meditations.

Sattva (sattvic): One of the three gunas, this is the quality of purity and lightness. A yogic diet consists mainly of sattvic foods.

Sivananda: Teacher of Swami Vishnu-devananda and inspiration behind the International Sivananda Yoga Vedanta Centers.

Sea salt: Derived from the evaporation of seawater, this is high in many minerals, such as calcium, that are lacking in ordinary salt.

Swami: A person who has taken spiritual vows, much the same as a monk or nun.

Tapas: Sanskrit term for "austerity" as a means of strengthening the mind. Many yogis fast or put restrictions on their eating habits for the purpose of building up willpower.

Tahini: Sesame seed paste, high in vitamin E and many minerals. It is very tasty and can be used in a variety of ways. Tahini is sold in most health-food stores. If you can't find it, peanut butter may be substituted.

Tamari: A form of soy sauce that has been made by a natural rather than a chemical process. It is cultured in much the same way as yogurt and contains many important minerals, but it is high in salt (although not as high as soy sauce) and should be used in moderation. If unavailable, use soy sauce.

Tamas (tamasic): One of the three gunas; this is the quality of darkness, inertia, and laziness. A person following a yogic diet would try to avoid tamasic foods, as well as situations and conditions that are tamasic.

Tempeh: A cultured soy food, sometimes with wheat, rice, millet, peanuts, or coconut. It is high in vitamin B12. Never eat tempeh raw; it needs thorough cooking.

Tofu (soybean curd): Weight for weight, a more effective protein than those from animal sources—and without the cholestrol or high calories. Fresh tofu can be kept refrigerated for up to a week in fresh water, which must be changed daily. Tofu is also available in dried form which has a different flavor from fresh. Dried tofu needs to be soaked before using. If you are planning to use tofu in an uncooked dish, steam it first for 2 to 3 minutes to kill any bacteria.

Vegans: People who do not eat any animal products, dairy foods, or honey.

Vegetarian cheese: Cheese made with plant rennet rather than animal rennet. Both hard and soft cheeses are available. Cheese made from soybeans, which is suitable for vegans, is also available.

Vishnu-devananda, Swami: Founder and guru of the International Sivananda Yoga Vedanta Centers.

Wakame: The most popular seaweed in Japan. It is a fine source of trace minerals and can be used to help soften the tough fibers of other vegetables. Rehydrated wakame looks like slippery spinach, and is a common ingredient in miso soup. Wakame combines well with noodles, rice, barley, and most vegetables.

Yeast flakes: Non-leavening "nutritional" yeast, high in B-vitamins. The flakes have a nutty, cheeselike flavor and can be sprinkled on any number of dishes for added nutritional impact. Available from most health-food stores, they are a good substitute for cheese.

Yogi: A person who practices physical and mental control to achieve a union of the individual soul with the Absolute.

Additional Reading

The Sivananda Companion to Yoga The Sivananda Yoga Center, Simon & Schuster
The New Vegetarian Colin Spencer, Viking
The Complete Illustrated Book of Yoga Swami Vishnu-devananda, Crown Publishers
Meditation and Mantras Swami Vishnu-devananda, OM Lotus Publishing
Hatha Yoga Pradipika Swami Vishnu-devananda, OM Lotus Publishing
Yoga Mind & Body The Sivananda Yoga Centre, Dorling Kindersley
The Life and Work of Swami Sivananda Vol 2: Health and Hatha Yoga Divine Life Society
Bliss Divine Swami Sivananda, Divine Life Society